HORMONE REPLACEMENT THERAPY: YES OR NO?

HOW TO MAKE AN INFORMED DECISION

about

ESTROGEN, PROGESTERONE, & OTHER STRATEGIES FOR DEALING WITH PMS, MENOPAUSE, & OSTEOPOROSIS

A new solution for the estrogen
replacement therapy dilemma

Betty Kamen, PhD

N⸻ ⸻⸻, California

D0951042

All of the facts in this book have been very carefully researched and have been drawn from the scientific literature. In no way, however, are any of the suggestions meant to take the place of advice given by physicians. Please consult a medical or health professional should the need for one be indicated.

Sixth Printing
Expanded & Updated
1997

Nutrition Encounter
PO Box 5847
Novato, CA 94948-5847
(415) 883-5154

Printed in the United States of America
First Printing   1993
Second Printing   1993
Third Printing   1995
Fourth Printing   1996
Fifth Printing   1996
Sixth Printing   1997

ISBN 0-944501-10-9

DEDICATED TO
John R. Lee, MD

ACKNOWLEDGMENTS

Research & Chart Development
    Paul Kamen

Support and Commitment
    Si Kamen
    Perle Kinney

Medical Expertise
    Serafina Corsello, MD
    Martin Milner, ND
    Michael Rosenbaum, MD
    Richard Kunin, MD
    Robert Atkins, MD
    Jerilynn Prior, MD
    Katherina Dalton, MD
    Raymond Peat, PhD

Feedback
    Bernice Goldmark, PhD
    Diana Hanssen

Editing
    Penny Post
    Theresa James Kamen

Cover Design
    Raylene Buehler

Graphic Arts
    New Vision Technologies, Inc.
    TechPool Studios
    ProArt Multi Ad Services
    T/Maker Company
    Wheeler Arts

CONTENTS

Figures

Tables

BOOKS & TAPES BY BETTY KAMEN, PhD

BOOKS

~ Kamut
  An Ancient Food for a Healthy Future
~ Everything You Always Wanted to Know About Potassium
  But Were Too Tired to Ask
~ New Facts About Fiber
  How Fiber Supplements Can Enhance Your Health
~ The Chromium Connection
  Diet & Supplement Strategy for Blood Sugar Control
~ Startling New Facts About Osteoporosis
  Why Calcium Alone Does Not Prevent Bone Disease
~ Germanium
  A New Approach to Immunity
~ Siberian Ginseng
  Up-to-Date Research on the Fabled Tonic Herb
~ Sesame—The Superfood Seed
  How It Can Add Vitality to Your Life
~ Nutrition In Nursing—The New Approach
  A Handbook of Nursing Science
~ Osteoporosis
  What It Is, How to Prevent It, How to Stop It
~ In Pursuit of Youth
  Everyday Nutrition for Everyone Over 35
~ Kids Are What They Eat
  What Every Parent Needs to Know About Nutrition
~ Total Nutrition for Breast-Feeding Mothers
~ Total Nutrition During Pregnancy
  How To Be Sure You and Your Baby Are Eating the
  Right Stuff

TAPES

~ Lessons in Nutrition: Table Talk Tapes (Audio)
  *Topics covered in this landmark series: Supplements, Food & Immunity,
  Antioxidants (OPCs or Pycnogenol), Memory, Osteoporosis, Remedies.*
~ Locker Room Logic: For Men Only
  Preventing & Reversing Prostate Problems
~ Hormone Replacement Therapy
  Audio & Video Tapes

Betty Kamen is an award-winning photojournalist with graduate degrees in psychology and nutrition education. She is an internationally-known lecturer, radio/TV host, and author of many major books, hundreds of articles, and tapes on various aspects of health and nutrition. For many years, she hosted Nutrition 57 on WMCA in New York, Nutrition Dialogue on SPN Cable Network, and Nutrition Watch on KNBR in San Francisco.

FOREWORD

Hormone Replacement Therapy: Yes or No? is a profoundly valuable educational resource—a reference that clearly and effectively educates women about their own hormones and body chemistry.

In the many years of treating women with natural progesterone and lifestyle changes for management of PMS and menopause, I searched far and wide for a definitive reference for patients—one that is thorough, up to date, and in language the general public can understand. Dr. Kamen's book is the arrival of that resource. Finally, women can have the information, tools, and resources needed to make informed decisions about their own endocrine balance.

A multiplicity of commonly-held fallacies are replaced with facts. These include the use of natural progesterone as an alternative to progestins and the integration of progesterone therapy into an existing estrogen therapy program.

The book invites the general public to sit down and enjoy a reading interlude that cannot help but foster a deep conviction in one's inherent self-healing abilities.

So hold on to your seats and get ready for an eye-opening experience into the truth surrounding hormone replacement therapy!

Martin Milner, ND
> *Medical Director, Center for Natural Medicine,*
> > *Portland, Oregon*
> *Associate Professor of Cardiovascular and Pulmonary*
> > *Medicine at National College of Naturopathic*
> > *Medicine*

AUTHOR'S NOTES:
VALIDATING THE CONCEPTS

More than 2,000 years ago, Hippocrates associated the consumption of high-fiber foods with better elimination. But the world didn't pay much attention until Denis Burkitt, MD, made the same "revolutionary" statement in 1980.

Why did it take more than two millennia to get from observation to acceptance to practice? Part of the reason is the natural lag that exists between research and application. Part of the reason is the "be-not-the-first-to-try-the-new" paradigm. And part of the reason may be inexplicable human behavior. Sometimes it takes twenty centuries, but the average lag time from initial reporting of concepts to general acceptance is currently 40 to 75 years—in spite of our high-tech disbursement of information.

It is gratifying to me to reflect on ideas that I have presented for almost five decades, and then to find that my conclusions (and those of other researchers like myself) have been validated years later. *The information presented in this book has already demonstrated the same history.*

I've been asked, time and again, what prompted me to write this book. The answer is: CONFUSION. As I lectured around the country, more and more women were asking about hormone replacement therapy: Should they take the synthetic drugs their doctors were advocating? Was it okay to start before they had any symptoms? What about the risks? What about the risks of NOT taking the drugs? How long should they stay on the drugs? Should they take the drugs if their mothers or sisters had breast cancer? If *they* had breast cancer? What about osteoporosis? What about heart protection? What about the new information on Alzheimer's disease?

Well, I had always believed that healthy women do not suffer from PMS, menopausal symptoms, or osteoporosis—ever. When I approached menopause more than twenty years ago, I was determined to be an example of this conviction. I studied the folk lore of herbs reported to keep women in "balance." After all, wasn't it true that if these remedies hadn't worked, they would not have stood the test of time?

Along with these herbs, I continued to consume the best possible foods. Now I understand why I never experienced *a single hot flash or day of discomfort.*

I decided to write a book about the advantages and disadvantages of the synthetic protocol, and offer a similar scenario for natural remedies. But things don't always turn out the way we expect. By the time I finished my research, I had come to three very startling conclusions:
(1) The side effects of taking synthetic estrogen and progestins are far greater than most people had ever realized, and that includes our medical community.
(2) Believe it or not, we simply do not need any more estrogen.
(3) There is a safe and easy remedy for most of these problems, one that doesn't require major lifestyle change. My personal experience predated the importance of progesterone. Nor did I know about an extract of a tuber containing progesterone-like activity (the Mexican wild yam).

So if you want a book that presents the pros and cons of both methods of assistance, this is not the one to read. Combining the wisdom of the ages with new information has been the focal point of much of my writing—especially of the details presented here. This book contains specifics about the significance of progesterone *and* the use of time-honored herbs for women's health.

Now the serendipity! Until recently, a preparation containing wild yam extract and progesterone was sold through professional sources only. An independent formulator used the research in my book to assemble newer products, adding herbal extracts I discuss in these pages. The synergy of these ingredients has produced remarkable success. The products are so safe, they are available to the public without prescription. (Needless to say, the best approach is to have guidance from physicians who are nutrition oriented.)

I have had the privilege of traveling all over the country to give presentations on the subject. This has given me the opportunity to talk to an endless number of practitioners and to hundreds of women—learning what has worked and what hasn't. I am convinced more than ever that hormones are not needed in high doses to be effective, and that adding specific herbs is extremely beneficial. When one aspect of health breaks down (i.e., hormone metabolism), you can be sure that other areas of health also decline.

The stories I have been hearing are awesome and come from men as well. A chiropractor reported that his libido returned to normal within two weeks. It had dropped to zero because of high blood pressure medication. (There is now a product for men that includes, in addition to the progesterone, several prostate-protective herbs.)

SCIENCE BY PRESS RELEASE:
The greatest problem we face is *science by press release*. The widespread "news" that estrogen therapy helps to prevent Alzheimer's disease is a case in point. If you examine the research, you will note that one study found a protective effect, another did not, and a third found the results inconclusive. But let's give the benefit of the doubt, and

assume that estrogen does offer protection from this disease, helping to prevent short-term memory loss. Does this mean that when we develop cancer (because we are on synthetic hormones), we will remember our pain and misery better? We know that steroids affect neuronal enzymatic pathways. Why not the safer steroid, *natural progesterone*?

Worse, when the stories extolling the benefits of drugs wind up on the front pages of our newspapers, on radio, and on TV, the public is usually unaware that only small sections of a study may be publicized by high-powered Madison Avenue PR firms, representing companies that often have a financial interest. The details of the article may even contradict the headliine, but only the headline information is repeated on national news. And when an article refuting these conclusions appears in the journals, there is no mention of this at all in the media. We call this **"Science by Press Release."**

Many of us have sacrificed our sense of control when it comes to making decisions about hormone replacement therapy. That's okay—if that's our choice—provided we don't forfeit our health as well. High technology should help us to understand our bodies, not be a force for attaining artificial and unnatural metabolism.

No book I have ever written has attracted as much attention from our more conservative medical community. Women tell me they give this book to their physicians, doctors call me with questions, and many practitioners keep the book on hand for their patients. Natural progesterone has lived up to its prophesy! Those physicians who put this successful therapy in place are to be commended. Lucky are their patients.

Betty Kamen

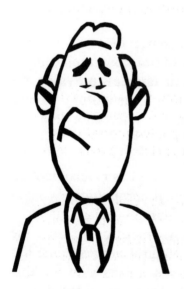
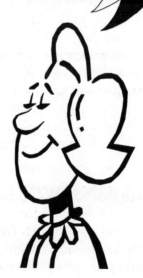

THE "HEALTHY-USER" SYNDROME

Articles on the hazards of postmenopausal hormone therapy are beginning to appear in prestigious medical journals. Even more noteworthy than citing the risks for HRT, are these comments in *New England Journal of Medicine* (1997, June19;336:1769-75):

> Observational studies have reported reduced mortality among women taking hormones, but many of the studies have had methodologic flaws that limit firm conclusions. Women for whom estrogen is prescribed are often healthier initially, and those who continue to take hormones tend to be free of disease. For example, women in whom cancer is diagnosed, often stop taking hormones. Thus, lower mortality among hormone users may be attibuted erroneously to the hormone istelf.

> The apparent benefit for coronary heart disease disappears within five years of stopping use, and there is little decrease for women at low risk of heart disease. Nor is there increasing benefit of hormones with increasing duration of use....Expected mortality advantages are, in part, offset by the risk of breast cancer.

> Women discontinue hormone use when symptoms of a fatal disease develop. This must reflect the selection of healthy women for estrogen therapy, a potential "healthy-user"effect. Postmenopausal estrogen probably acts as a late-stage growth promoter. We know many ways to lower risk of coronary disease, but few to lower the risk of breast cancer.

Similar articles have appeared in other journals. Read on!

The *British Medical Journal* (1997, Jul 19;315:149-53) cites that the pooled data of clinical trials "do not support the notion that postmenopausal hormone therapy prevents cardiovascular events." These researchers looked at 22 trials involving 4,124 women. They conclude:

> There have been hundreds of trials studying the impact of hormones on various physiological phenomena, laboratory values, osteoporosis, symptoms, or various health problems, but few fully report adverse effects....In many trials, women were lost to follow up, and even more trials gave no data on reasons or numbers of drop outs or losses. Most trials had selected only healthy women. Therefore, the effects of postmenopausal therapy on sick women cannot be inferred from these results....Carcinogenic effects or slow tumor promotion may take years or decades to show up. (These studies were not long-term.) Studies failed to report adverse effects fully, if at all.

Additional reports:
New England Jnl of Medicine, 1997, June 19; 336:1821
Progestins may diminish the apparently cardioprotective effect of estrogen therapy.

Maturitas 1996 Oct;259(2):107-14
The protective effect of estrogen against cardiovascular diseases in women disappears after menopause.

American Jnl of Epidemiology 1996 May 15;143:971-8
Women who elect to use ERT have a better cardiovascular risk factor profile prior to the use of ERT than do women who subsequently do not use this treatment during menopause, which supports the hypothesis that part of the apparent benefit associated with the use of ERT is due to preexisting characteristics of women who use ERT.

Beware of the "healthy-user" syndrome.

INTRODUCTION

SERAFINA CORSELLO, MD

As I was pondering the necessity of writing a book about the hormonal problems of women—from the cradle to the golden years—my dear friend Betty Kamen seized the keyboard and produced this most comprehensive, magnificent review of the physiology and pathology of the female reproductive cycle.

Betty Kamen is one of the most prolific medical writers. Her nutritional background gives her the authority to write cogently about the subjects she covers. As usual, she provides an incredible number of references which can be used by the reader for further research. Betty's books are well-indexed and well-documented. She arrives at brilliant medical deductions that I find very enlightening.

Betty proposes the theory that until the turn of the century very few women suffered the dreadful consequences of hormonal derangement, primarily because of their judicious diet. This is certainly true.

Betty suggests (as I do) that there has been a well-known biased attitude in regard to women's problems. As a physician and a woman, I have had to recognize the subtle discriminatory attitudes that have been so pervasive in the medical field. Until very recently, the male-dominated medical establishment felt much more comfortable relegating women's hormonal problems to the insane asylum, rather than to the benches of biomedical research.

I believe that the heightened interest in research into female reproductive functions will continue because of the economic issues relating to it. In the next twenty years approximately forty million women will enter menopause. No medical establishment, and certainly no pharmaceutical industry, will ignore such a large population with its potential for so much economic return.

Most of this research, however, focuses solely on estrogen replacement therapy. Very little has been done regarding safe, nontoxic alternatives—which this book so eloquently describes. Unless menopause once again becomes an *uneventful stage of life*, we will be troubled by a plethora of dreadful medical consequences.

We women will be spending *one-third* of our lives in a postmenopausal state. We need to be able to function without the threat of poorly managed menopause and its harmful consequences.

As a postmenopausal woman, I have had to deal personally with the reality of estrogen replacement therapy. At age fifty-two, when I experienced the abrupt onset of insomnia which would not permit me to function at the high level to which I was accustomed, I turned to the "quick fix"—*hormonal replacement therapy*, which includes estrogen and synthetic progestin.

At age fifty-four, I awoke one morning with an ominous mass in my breast. I had to discontinue the hormones immediately but was faced with the necessity of finding a substitute for them. There was no book such as this to guide me, so I went to the library and read all I could find on the subject of natural, traditional, and Eastern interventions for hot flashes and insomnia—the two most common symptoms related to these later years.

My newly-found knowledge forged the basis of my interest in *natural* replacement therapy. I have since used these interventions on myself and my patients, with great results. Betty's book provides ample tools to assist women in the important task of recognition of the early signs of menopause and what to do about them. And so much of this information pertains to PMS as well.

One of the first markers of hormone imbalance is irritability. Women often report being besieged by a loosely-defined sense of malaise. They say, "I'm just not the same." In some cases, they fall into a state of bewilderment and depression. These are the women who populate the welcoming couches of psychoanalysts in search of elusive answers.

Another change occurs in the quality and/or quantity of the menstrual flow. All of a sudden a cycle will skip, and the next one may be frighteningly heavy with clots and pain. *Until there is ovarian failure, the diagnosis is in the art of empathic listening.*

I have had to recognize that as sympathetic as I thought I had always been, I became a more sensitive, receptive antenna to my patients' subtle problems when I myself went through the experience. Life is the best teacher, but, as our experiences with homogeneous support groups have taught us, this does not mean that only people who experience problems can treat them. It only means that they may be able to do it better.

At a time when the body is going through fluctuations of estrogen and progesterone, the sense of instability is understandably worse. This comprehensive book gives wonderful suggestions that can help avoid the unpleasantness associated with changing hormone ratios.

Unencumbered by the responsibilities of young women—fear of pregnancy and care of our children—we can, in later years, set out to become what we really are. Post-menopausal liberation can lead to a splendid valley of achievements. My dear friend Betty is a perfect example of this model.

If one can reach the menopausal zest, it can be one of the most rewarding stages of life. As Betty suggests, one "cashes in at the end what one has saved at the beginning."

Unfortunately for us, the beginning may go as far back as our prenatal phase. One of my greatest joys is the treatment of infertile women, who, through natural methodology, then become fertile. These women continue to eat well, take adequate nutrients, have a joyous attitude, and deliver what I call "super babies." These babies, if they continue to take good care of themselves throughout their lives, will have none of the problems associated with menopausal "storms."

I have seen patients in whom menopausal symptoms become worse when they take synthetic progestins, as prescribed during hormone replacement therapy. This has convinced me, more than anything else, to put myself and my patients on the kind of program that Betty outlines.

Women with severe PMS can count on difficulties at the end of the road. Treating PMS naturally prevents the difficulty later in life.

By writing such a cogent and comprehensive book on the natural management of all female hormonal problems, Betty Kamen has given a new lease on life to thousands of women. As a clinician, I can attest to the fact that diet, attitude, and natural interventions do make an *enormous* difference. Since PMS is marked by a dysfunction in progesterone and vitamin B_6 metabolism (among other nutrient factors), intervening with natural progesterone and with micronutrients has a tremendous therapeutic value. Vitamin B_6, as explained in this book, participates in the enhancement of proper estrogen metabolism. It is important to understand that nature likes balance, and that nutrients are co-dependent.

Fortunately, Betty emphasizes this concept and provides many nontoxic tools. She teaches us how to balance *all* elements of life. She has succeeded in giving a compendium of events that can lead to a safe hormonal voyage. Betty takes us step by step through that journey, illustrating how everything works. The goal is to achieve an easy transition. The result is the attainment of postmenopausal zest.

Congratulations, Betty, and congratulations to your readers.

Serafina Corsello, MD
Director, Corsello Centers
New York, New York; Huntington, New York
Member, National Institutes of Health, ad hoc committee of
the Office of Alternative Medicine

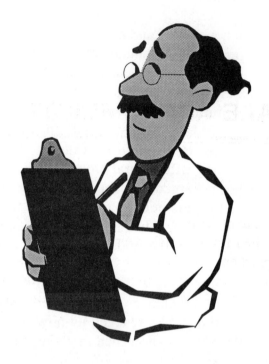

You want to know if you should go on hormone replacement therapy? Well, yes and no. But don't quote me!

I

FEMALE AND AFFLICTED

HOW IT IS, HOW IT WAS, HOW IT COULD BE

When I began my research for this book, I was astounded to learn that the first scientific description of what we now call PMS, or premenstrual syndrome, did not appear until 1931. Difficulties relating to menstruation were then referred to as premenstrual tension—and even that designation is a product of relatively modern-day classification. The initials PMS did not became part of the medical (and popular) lexicon until 1953, when Katherina Dalton and Raymond Greene published a paper called "The Premenstrual Syndrome." At long last, PMS was recognized as a collection of loosely-related symptoms—described in the medical literature.

Why didn't it happen before 1953? Hadn't half the population of the world suffered, more or less, with PMS every month of every year for the entire history of the human species? Are we to believe that very few women suffered from PMS before 1931? Or that the variety of symptoms had never been correlated and listed before 1953? After all, hadn't the symptoms of many other significant disorders been recorded with explicit detail over the centuries?

Certainly there's always been a male bias in academic medical research. But even making allowances for possible neglect, it seems incredible that a problem so universal should have received so little attention. Similarly, the focus on the ever-increasing incidence of breast cancer and on the difficulties related to menopause are very recent developments. Even osteoporosis was unknown terminology outside the medical profession just a few years ago; *now it's a household word.*

Had these disorders been ignored? Or did doctors have completely different names or different diagnoses for them? What was going on?

The answer is discouragingly simple. The physicians who cared for our grandmothers and great-grandmothers weren't very concerned about PMS, osteoporosis, menopausal problems, or breast cancer *because our grandmothers and great-grandmothers weren't very concerned about them, either.* Menstrual and menopausal problems just didn't come up that often among our naturally nourished ancestors. Yet in this century we have come to accept these irregularities as part of being female—a universal constant of the gender. I seriously question this assumption. Truly healthy women *do not* suffer from these diseases—ever!

Before you dismiss me as a hopeless nutritional idealist, let me add that the conditions of "well-nourished" and "healthy" are admittedly elusive goals that very few women fully achieve in North America. We are all under continuous assault from pollution, exercise deprivation, stress, and the abysmally poor quality of what we have come to regard as "normal" food—not to mention the effects of poor lighting, environmental chemicals, and the strained ergonomics of the typical indoor workplace.

Compare our current environment with that of only a few generations ago when the daily routine was full of physical activity; the air was clean; indoor smoke was rare; chemical solvents were unheard of; devices that produce stray electromagnetic fields had yet to be invented.

Another major difference concerns our food. Once upon a time, food was full of nutrients and free of pesticides. It was locally produced and genetically unaltered. Most importantly, it was fresh, and it wasn't junk—no soda, ice cream, donuts, potato chips, or pop tarts. Hardly any sugar and not much salt. There were lots of vegetables eaten in season along with freshly killed meat or freshly caught fish (when it was available). Food was preserved for winter without benefit of a chemical engineer.

> **Before World War II, processed food was the exception, not the rule.**

You probably still think I'm a hopeless idealist when it comes to food, diet, and health. "Sure," you must be thinking, "as if I can turn back the clock a hundred years and be magically free of all my health problems."

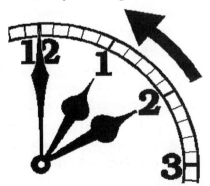

We all know we can't turn the clock back.
(We don't want to!)

Even if we were to swear off the supermarket, the car, and the office forever and walk into the woods to eat nothing but just-caught fish, just-killed meat (eating most of it uncooked), and freshly picked fruits and vegetables, we could never return to the optimal health of people who have lived like that all of their lives. Damage has been done, beginning with our parents' (and possibly our grandparents') lifestyles before we were conceived. *Nutrition crosses generation lines.*

And even if we could turn that clock back, would we really want to give up the convenience of our postindustrial, high-tech lifestyle in pursuit of that last vaguely tangible increment of optimal health?

We are left with serious compromises. Although we still have much to learn, we do know a lot about menopause, osteoporosis, PMS, and breast cancer, and there are accepted treatments for all these problems. But there are major differences among the various forms of doctoring and management. Some remedies short-circuit natural healing mechanisms, while others enhance them. Most doctor-prescribed treatments are interventionist—they do nothing more than suppress symptoms, never getting to causes. Worse, they interfere with our body's natural methods for correcting imbalances.

"Recommendations for hormone replacement therapy for women who do not have symptoms are currently not justified."
Eur J Obstet Gyneco Reprod Biol 1997;71:205.

"Estrogen therapy is associated with a large increase in risk of endometrial cancer, an association that almost certainly is a causal one."
Maturitas 1996; 23:235.

WHAT THIS BOOK IS ABOUT

This book examines today's strategies for dealing with PMS, menopause, and osteoporosis, and suggests ways for you to decide on personal action in these areas. Estrogen therapy in the treatment and prevention of osteoporosis is discussed, as well as natural progesterone as an alternative—plus reasons for the use of certain herbs and food supplements. My views spring from: (1) clinical experience; (2) a broad range of interviews with medical professionals; (3) intensive research of published literature.

I want to share with you:

> Facts and fallacies about PMS, menopause, and osteoporosis
> Advantages and disadvantages of estrogen therapy with emphasis on increasing evidence demonstrating how and why this therapy is harmful
> Advantages and disadvantages of adding synthetic progestins to hormone therapy
> Advantages of adding natural progesterone to hormone therapy
> The rationale for using natural progesterone *transdermally* (that is, entering through the skin)
> The rationale for adding hormone-regulating herbs to this therapy
> The basis for including certain food supplements
> The justification for specific food cautions

After extensive examination of all sides of the issues, I have formed fairly strong conclusions. You will find in these pages that I frequently take positions advocating specific courses of action. Although there is certainly no shortage of controversy, I would be doing you a disservice if I were to avoid passing along my conclusions, opinions, and even hunches.

The sources of the prestigious medical research that I have scrutinized and the details of my interviews with the clinicians—all of which helped bring me to these conclusions—are cited throughout this book.

Simply stated, I am an advocate of using a plant extract containing progesterone-like activity, plus a small amount of the natural progesterone hormone itself, mixed in a cream base with specific herbs. I have now been witness to endless success stories from women and their practitioners, the result of using this treatment as an alternative to the more traditional hormone therapy. You should know that I didn't start out with this view. Before my research, I was more inclined to oppose any therapy that presumes to improve on nature's own balance of hormones. But without intending to, I assembled a compelling case for this natural product. It has been difficult to find a single informed source that has anything negative to say about such a mode of treatment. I'm convinced that this is the way to go, and, hopefully, you will be, too.

Impressive evidence now validates beyond a doubt that progesterone, progesterone-like extracts, and certain herbs can correct a deficiency which is proving to be the *real* cause of PMS, the *real* cause of menopausal symptoms, the *real* cause of osteoporosis.

Should *you* start using this combination of natural progesterone and hormone-balancing herbs and extracts in cream form? Should *you* do this instead of taking the hormone therapy your doctor may be prescribing? Should *you* proceed without your physician's full cooperation? These are the questions answered here. But you are not going to get off easy if you decide to opt for better health. The use of natural progesterone and hormone-regulating herbs, while far safer than alternatives, are still an intervention to be applied with knowledge and care.

Furthermore, this combination of special substances is only part of the solution, at best. You probably already know that if you want to enjoy optimal health, you'll have to give up a few fast-held, fast-food habits. You may also be surprised to discover that you'll have to reverse a few practices you thought were healthful. In fact, to be totally free of annoying discomforts, some of you may have to make what you would consider substantial sacrifices in your nutritional lifestyle. The point is that such a goal is entirely possible, regardless of your health status.

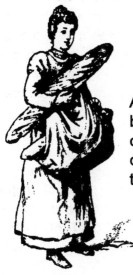

Are we talking about turning back the clock again? No, we can't retreat to the nineteenth century. Again—we don't want to.

Fortunately, we are in a position to pick and choose knowledge of the past and present, and to project future choices based on this wisdom. If we are successful, we'll be able to give PMS, osteoporosis, and menopausal symptoms as little regard as the women and physicians of generations ago. Even more exciting is the potential to wipe out breast cancer, now recognized as a totally avoidable disease.

Please note that the term *natural progesterone* is redundant. Progesterone infers that the hormone is natural, but I use the redundancy to stress the point.

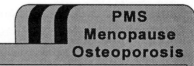

MEMOS

➢ About 90 percent of American women have some type of menstrual complaint. Typical comments:

> "Once a month, I feel as though 50 boy scouts tie knots in my groin."
> "Once a month, a butterfly collection is let loose in my stomach."
> "Once a month, the Music Man's 76 trombones parade around in my head."
> "Yesterday, I spent a year doing routine office work."

➢ Tribal rituals welcoming young girls to womanhood at the start of menstruation were very happy occasions, including song, laughter, and dance. It was considered a sacred time during which women were not to be disturbed. Menstrual taboos were created to protect women.

➢ In more primitive societies today, menstruation is not associated with a syndrome, and fewer women complain of cramps or discomfort than in our advanced culture.[1]

➢ Many physicians (and their patients) confirm that switching to nutrient-dense diets results in the disappearance of PMS.

MEMOS

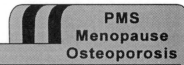

PMS
Menopause
Osteoporosis

➤ Case Western Reserve Medical School discusses the good-health practices of a tribal South African group that is totally free of menopausal symptoms.[2]

➤ The French *Journal of Obstetrics and Gynecology* reminds us that the nutritional demands for certain nutrients are high during menopause and that the consequences of deficiencies are hormonal disturbances.[3]

➤ Not all postmenopausal women develop osteoporosis, as pointed out in the German publication, *Wiener Medizinisch Wochenschrift.*[4]

➤ The *Annual Review of Nutrition* noted that when *diet*, physical activity, cigarette smoking, and alcohol consumption are modified, the usual risks associated with menopause are reduced.[5]

➤ There are cultures in the world where words for PMS or hot flash simply do not exist because the problems don't exist..

➤ After two generations of acculturation to American ways, Japanese women become subject to our same afflictions.

➤ According to a 1996 report, patient acceptance of standard cyclic HRT has been poor.

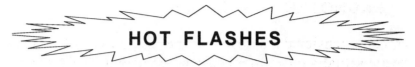

HOT FLASHES

➢ One of every six white North American women will have a hip fracture during her lifetime—the most important cause of ill health and death among older people. One in three develops osteoporosis.

New England Jnl of Medicine, 1995[6]
Zentralblatt fur Gynakologie, 1994[7]
International Jnl of Clinical Pharmacology,
Therapy, and Toxicology, 1992[8]

➢ Osteoporosis is expensive and disabling; getting it to some degree is almost certain.

Optimal Health Guidelines, 1993[9]

➢ Most "new" diseases are caused by an external agent. We continue to inflict new diseases on ourselves due to environmental changes or medical intervention.

Lancet, 1993[10]

➢ Recognizing a new disease may be delayed until it is widespread enough and medicine is ready to receive it. Physicians today are confronted with new diseases and mysteriously rampant infections.

Lancet, 1993[11]
New England Jnl of Medicine, 1995[12]

UPDATES

Maturitas 1996 May;23(Suppl):S37-45
Intake of both estradiol compounds and conjugated estrogens increase the risk of breast cancer 1.5- to 2-fold. The addition of progestins does not reduce the duration-risk relationship. The level of risk for endometrial cancer is about 10-fold after 10 or more years of intake.

Cancer Causes & Control 1996 Nov;7(6):575-80
Women who have discontinued estrogen therapy may retain a small increased risk of endometrial cancer for a long period of time.

~~ ENDNOTES ~~ *A Fantasy...*

Three-dimensional movies—the ones that make us feel that we are actually *on* a roller coaster—contribute to a fantasy I've had for years. I have wished we could be placed inside our very own bodies, perhaps through high-tech simulation, something not unlike a computerized virtual-reality sensory jumpsuit. Or maybe even with an old-fashioned Aladdin's lamp. Instead of roller-coaster whirlings coursing through our heads and stomachs, as in the movies of my youth, we would encounter a visual sensing of hormonal happenings. *We would have a direct view of the magic of metabolism.*

We could then be witness to the power, the authority, the wonder of our hormones *while their actions are in progress.* We would know just how they work and how they affect our health—for better or for worse.

Since neither our computers nor our science (nor our magic) have reached that level of sophistication, we must resort to more conventional modes of learning. The next section explains some of what we know about hormones—knowledge that may help us make our decisions about hormone replacement therapy.

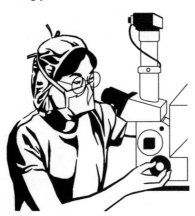

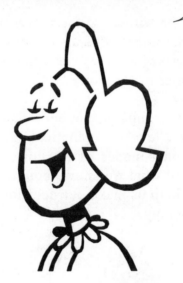

2

WHAT IS A HORMONE?

WHAT HORMONES DO

We're all familiar with sex hormones. But hormones control a lot more of our body's functions than sex. Hormones are secreted by glands (such as your pancreas, adrenal, thyroid, and ovaries) in very small quantities, usually into your bloodstream. As hormones journey around, they activate, control, or direct the actions of other organs and tissues. No wonder the word hormone stems from the Greek *hormaein*, which means *to excite*.

Like foods, hormones are consumed as energy and are not produced as by-products of metabolic processes. They are specifically aimed at controlling other actions in your body, often at a location far from where they are produced. Your body doesn't physically direct a hormone to a particular tissue or organ unless the target is right next to the gland producing the hormone (or is producing the hormone itself). A hormone travels until it is recognized by a receptor shaped to fit, the way pieces of a jigsaw puzzle fit together.

Hormones help some of your cells create protective "coats of armor." They instruct molecular switches to turn on or off. They mandate immune processes to grapple with invaders, and charge receptors to stoke fires that require more fuel. They are responsible for glands inducing *differentiation*, prodding a cell which appears to be able to turn into *anything* during the fetal stage, to turn into *something very specific* years, even decades, later.

FIGURE 1

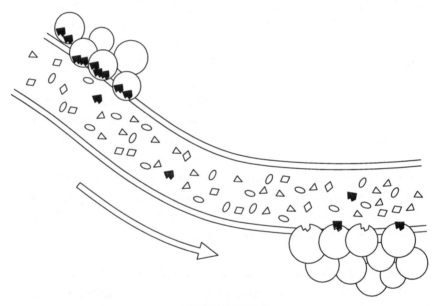

HORMONES:
FROM GLAND TO TARGET ORGAN

A small concentration of a hormone can affect tissue at a remote location. The circles at upper left represent cells in a hormone-producing gland. Hormones are represented by the black particles. The hormone enters the bloodstream and will only exit when encountering a matching receptor, as represented by the circles at lower right. Other hormones are not affected by this receptor—they just don't "fit."

Hormones generally spread out evenly through your blood-stream, much like a broadcast radio signal. Only certain cells of certain organs or tissues have their chemical receptors "tuned in" to respond to the effects of that particular hormone. (See Figure 1 on page 22.)

It's amazing how few hormone molecules are required to produce a major effect. At the top end of the range, there is only one hormone molecule for every *fifty billion* molecules in your blood plasma. At the low end of the concentration scale, there may be one hundred times fewer hormone molecules—one in every *five zillion*. That's five thousand billion! This is comparable to one crystal of salt in a large swimming pool. *Keep this in mind when you consider intervening with the use of synthetic hormones in your own body.*

Functionally, hormones can be divided into four categories. There are hormones to control:
> (1) Energy production and storage
> (2) Water and salt metabolism
> (3) Growth
> (4) Sexual and reproductive actions

Of course, there's a certain degree of overlap. If it were not for the effects of progesterone and estrogen on the integrity of your bones, for example, you would have fewer reasons to be reading this book. The multiple interrelationships between various hormones and other nutrients make the subject interesting—but also create controversy in attempts to maintain optimal health. And it can be especially confusing for those whose physicians recommend hormone replacement therapy in *anticipation* of trouble. Many doctors sincerely believe that certain difficulties are inescapable with age. Fortunately, others do not share this view and have demonstrated its fallacy.

Your glands manufacture hormones from:
  (1) Amino acids
  (2) Proteins or peptides
  (3) Cholesterol

Hormones made from cholesterol are called *steroid* hormones—the category discussed here. We often associate the word steroid with the huge muscles adorning men on the covers of sports magazines, just as we associate the word cholesterol with the "bad" fatty substance found in most animal-derived food (that nasty heart-disease and arteriosclerosis accomplice). But steroid hormones play many vital and beneficial roles in human metabolism. *Cholesterol serves as an important building block for necessary hormones.*

Cholesterol's role in heart disease is actually somewhat indirect, and it hardly deserves the terrible reputation it has acquired over the last few decades. Interestingly, cholesterol is produced in almost every cell in your body. Your liver spews it out in especially large quantities.

The cholesterol in whole foods (in fresh eggs or pure meat, for example) has still not been proved significantly responsible for contributing to the cholesterol buildup that damages arteries.

Dietary cholesterol itself is an innocent bystander, while many other factors contribute to excessive cholesterol buildup and arteriosclerosis. Among these factors are:

  ➢ Processed fats exposed to heat, light, air, and time
  ➢ Nutrient deficiencies, including vitamin B_6
  ➢ Stress

Figure 2 on page 26 demonstrates a diagram of a cholesterol molecule and some of the other hormone molecules made from it. Notice how much of each molecule is identical in each representation. The similar part of each of these cholesterol molecules is referred to as the *17-carbon backbone*.

Now notice the relatively subtle modifications of this cholesterol backbone. The minor variations identify the hormone.

> The difference between testosterone and estradiol (one type of estrogen) is simply the addition of one hydrogen atom. When one notch on a key is just a little bit different, it opens a completely different lock.

Another factor that distinguishes steroid hormones is that they generally cannot be stored inside the cells of the glands that manufacture them. Rather, they are released immediately into your bloodstream as soon as they are produced.

> Since steroid hormones are made from cholesterol, it's important to have an ample supply of cholesterol available at all times. Also crucial: an adequate provision of the nutrients producing the enzymes necessary for the cholesterol synthesis. This is one of many examples of the interdependence of nutrient-biological processes.

FIGURE 2

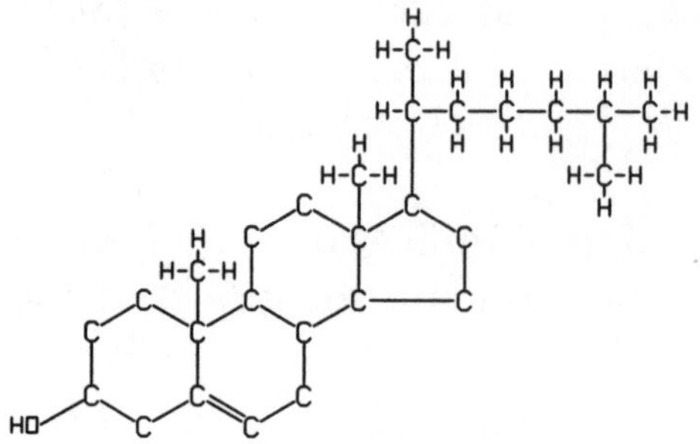

CHOLESTEROL

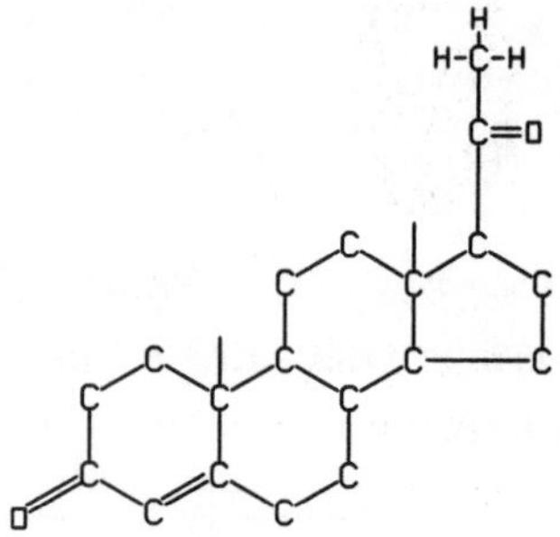

PROGESTERONE

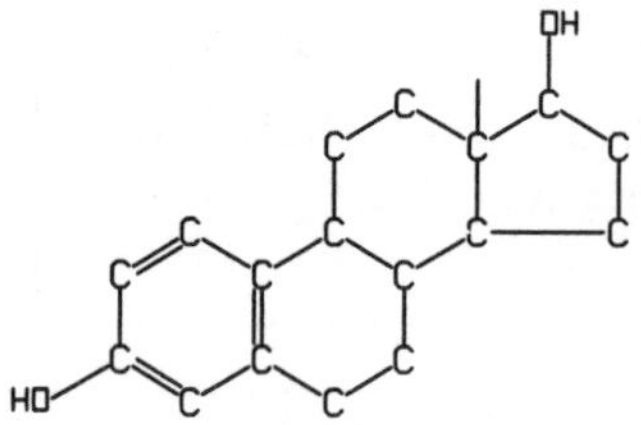

ESTRADIOL

(an estrogen)

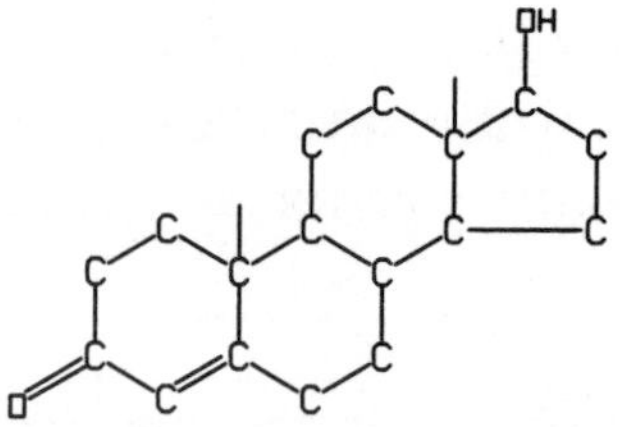

TESTOSTERONE

(an androgen)

THE CHOLESTEROL MOLECULE AND THREE STEROID HORMONES MADE FROM IT

This represents the cholesterol molecule and three steroid hormones that can be manufactured from it by your adrenal cortex. Notice how little difference there is between the androgen *testosterone* and the estrogen *estradiol*.

WHAT HAPPENS WHEN YOU EAT HORMONES?

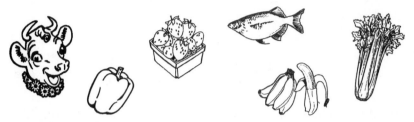

Meat, fish, and even fruits and vegetables contain all the hormones and enzymes used to regulate their life processes when they were living organisms—before they became food. If their blend of chemical signals suddenly becomes mixed with *your* hormones and enzymes, the result would be disastrous—like trying to run a complicated machine with the wrong set of instructions. So immediately after hormones are digested in your small intestines, they pass through your liver, which is pretty smart: *Your liver helps you get rid of these unnecessary hormones.*

One of your liver's most important jobs is to break down foreign hormones or keep them out of your bloodstream by returning them to your digestive tract.

There's an interesting design feature here: Your liver returns the unwanted hormones to your digestive tract at the entrance to your small intestines, where they could get reabsorbed! It's like placing the sewage outlet up-river from where the town gets its drinking water. Did nature miss something at this juncture? No! This method of disposal works because the hormones, *first time around*, are converted by your liver into water-soluble forms. They now bind with other substances, making them difficult to get absorbed through your intestines the *second time around*.

In fact, the materials that cause the hormones to return to your digestive tract and render them *excretable,* may also act on newly ingested hormones on their first pass through your intestines. So some ingested hormones don't get absorbed even once! This process is called *first-pass liver removal.*

We have, then:
    (1) The removal of ingested hormones by your liver
    (2) The chemical environment of your intestines that makes hormone absorption difficult

Given these two factors, only a tiny fraction of dietary female hormones and enzymes normally make it into your bloodstream for general circulation.

Considering your body's sensitivity to very small quantities of hormones, it's easy to understand why first-pass hormone removal is an important function of your liver. But because of first-pass removal, administering hormones by mouth is wrought with complications.

The big breakthrough in oral contraception was the development of a form of hormones that could be absorbed readily by your digestive system, making the birth control pill a reality.

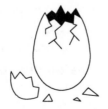

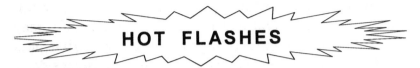

HOT FLASHES

➢ Dietary fiber in your diet affects the way prescribed estrogen will be metabolized in your liver.

Jnl of the Pakistan Medical Association, 1994[1]

➢ The impact of [synthetic] estrogen on bone metabolism is dependent on how the estrogen is administered.

Jnl of Bone and Mineral Research, 1992[2]

➢ The effects of different modes of estrogen administration have only recently been recognized.

Thrombosis Haemostasis, 1994[3]

➢ Controlled levels of estrogen are difficult because of first-pass liver metabolism.

Drugs, 1990[4]

➢ Blood concentrations of estrogen after similar doses vary—depending on the mode of administration.

Minerva Endocrinologica, 1989[5]

➢ Undesirable effects of estrogen are hard to avoid when estrogen is taken orally.

Drugs, 1990[6]

➢ Doses of estrogen must be adjusted to achieve desired levels.

Minerva Endocrinologica, 1989[7]

➢ The effectiveness of estrogen is dependent on the dosage and mode of application.

Zentralblatt fur Gynakologie, 1989[8]

➢ After oral application, estrogens always experience the first-pass effect.

Zentralblatt fur Gynakologie, 1989[9]

➢ Fourteen eggs a week do not influence coronary heart-disease risk.

American Jnl of Clinical Nutrition, 1992[10]

➢ After six weeks of extra egg consumption, serum HDL cholesterol increased by 10 percent (that's good!); the ratio of total cholesterol/HDL cholesterol did not change significantly (that's good, too!).

Jnl of Internal Medicine, 1994[11]

UPDATES

Journal of the National Cancer Institute, May 15, 1996
Women may be getting bad news when they don't need
to! Those on ERT are more likely to get a false positive
reading on a mammogram than other women. Estrogen is believed to increase the amount of dense tissue
in the breasts, making it more difficult to correctly identify abnormalities.

1996 Medical Tribune News Service
Thirty million American women who will reach menopause in the next two decades will consider hormone
replacement therapy, including supplemental estrogen
and sometimes progestin. Estrogen replacement has
been found to increase the risk of uterine cancer.

1996 Medical Tribune News Service
Women with irregular menstrual cycles or other gynecological problems may be at increased risk for chronic
fatigue syndrome (CFS), according to the American
Public Health Association. Abnormal production of estrogen may play a role in triggering CFS by somehow
altering the immune system. This may explain why more
women than men are affected by the condition. The government officially recognizes CFS as a medical condition.

Jnl of the Amer Medical Assoc 1996;276:1747-1751
If you are on ERT, one to two glasses of wine will result
in a three-fold increase in the level of estrogen circulating in your blood. Increased blood levels of estrogen
may heighten your risk of breast cancer. Estrogen levels of women on estrogen replacement begins to rise
within 10 minutes of taking a drink of alcohol.

It has been said that the control panel of
a space shuttle is not as complicated as the
"control panel" of our livers!

~~ ENDNOTES ~~ *The fantasy continues...*

We watch, wide-eyed, as hormones enter the fast-moving vehicle (our bloodstream) that transports substances vital to our lives. We hear the counter clicking away, chalking up the rounds—graphically demonstrating that every single minute, *one thousand four hundred and forty times a day*, our blood circles through our body. We are fascinated by the hormonal activity—endless processes taking place concurrently—a three-ring circus, and more.

Some of the work of creating hormones has been farmed out, produced elsewhere—not inside our bodies. These hormones are a little different from those assembled by our own "factories." We observe a synthetic hormone playing the field, accepted here, rejected there. We listen to conversations—one gland to another, one group of cells to another—discussing the differences of the material we have swallowed, either intentionally by prescription or inadvertently in our food. "Can't fool us," we hear them saying.

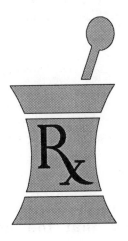

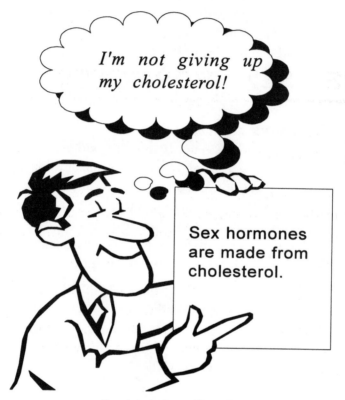

Reprinted from *New Facts About Fiber*
by Betty Kamen, Nutrition Encounter, 1991.

3

THE SEX HORMONES

TESTOSTERONE, ESTROGEN, AND PROGESTERONE

Testosterone, estrogen, and progesterone are hormones. More specifically, sex hormones. What? There are *three* sex hormones? In fact, there are several more, but these are the three principal sex hormones.

The word *testosterone* identifies a hormone made in the testes. The word *estrogen* comes from the Greek, meaning "producing frenzy." It has been suggested that the differences in the sources of terminology reflect the bias of the male researchers who coined the term estrogen in 1927.[1]

We normally use the words testosterone and estrogen as if they are male and female counterparts. But that's not exactly the way it is. Testosterone is one hormone of a general class of hormones called *androgens*. Androgens taken as a group, including testosterone, have the tissue-building and sex characteristics normally associated with the male sex hormone. *Estrogen*, unlike testosterone but like androgen, is the name for a class of hormones which includes several closely related substances associated with females. And both men and women produce androgens and estrogens!

So it's not really estrogen per se that produces many of the estrogen-related effects. When you read about estrogen and testosterone, understand that it's common to be a little loose with the jargon. For total clarity, let's summarize: Testosterone is only one of a broad class of hormones, the androgens. *Estrogen*, like *androgen* (but unlike *testosterone)*, also refers to an entire class of hormones. (See Figure 3 below.)

FIGURE 3

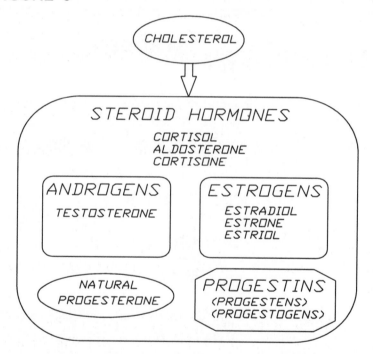

HOW CATEGORIES OF STEROID HORMONES ARE RELATED

Estrogens, androgens, and natural progesterone are steroid hormones—all made from cholesterol. Even though progestins are referred to as steroids, they do not occur naturally in human physiology.

Unfortunately, confusion abounds concerning the proper use of the term progesterone. Progesterone refers to one specific hormone—the natural one manufactured by your adrenal glands or ovaries. Progesterone is functionally related to (but *not* a member of) the class of synthetic hormones called *progestins*. Progestins may also be referred to as progestens, progestogens (also spelled progestegins in the medical literature), gestagens, or progestational agents.

Keep in mind that *all* progestins are synthetic hormones, closely resembling the progesterone hormone made in your body, but differing in significant ways. Just as the term "natural progesterone" is redundant, so the expression "synthetic progestin" is redundant.

The distinction between synthetic progestin and natural progesterone is extremely important. The term *progesterone treatment* is often used to describe the therapeutic administration of a synthetic progestin rather than the real thing, and is even confused by physicians! This is incorrect usage of the term. The difference between natural and synthetic progesterone is not unlike the difference between leather and vinyl car seats. They may even look somewhat the same, but just wait till you get into the car on a hot day!

Progesterone is the primary building block for all the other steroid hormones. This alone distinguishes natural progesterone from synthetic progestin, which is incapable of performing this function. The one similarity between synthetic and natural forms of this hormone is that they both promote endometrium secretion. Each can trigger uterine bleeding similar to menstrual flow. When this occurs with the use of natural progesterone, however, it is usually a needed "cleaning out" process, and rarely continues beyond a single cycle.[2]

Any substance produced by a human, an animal, or even a plant, cannot be patented unless its structure is molecularly altered or its use or function is changed. But a patent can be obtained for a hormone that varies from the natural. Does this explain the popularity of synthetic hormones promoted by drug companies? Would a board of directors allocate millions to develop and promote a product for hormone therapy if it could not get patent protection for the substance involved?

FIGURE 4

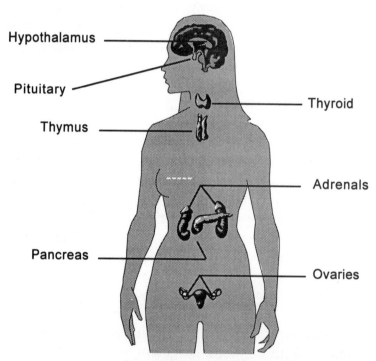

Hypothalamus

Pituitary

Thymus

Thyroid

Adrenals

Pancreas

Ovaries

MAJOR HORMONE-PRODUCING GLANDS

Different types of hormone-secreting cells make up the endocrine system, influenced in part by the nervous system. Hormones are varied. The female and male sex hormones (estrogens and testosterone) are all steroids.

BEHIND THE SCENES OF HORMONE PRODUCTION

Before puberty, your adrenals—the pyramid-shaped glands sitting on top of each kidney—are responsible for making all cholesterol-based, or steroid, sex hormones. (Your adrenal cortex is that part of each of your adrenal glands that actually makes the steroids.) Controlling this function is your pituitary, the tiny gland near the base of your brain—a gland so small it weighs no more than a paper clip.

Your pituitary, in turn, is regulated by your hypothalamus, the *master gland* which can almost be regarded as part of your brain. *This is the neurological link to steroid hormone production.* Messages from your brain are transmitted by way of your hypothalamus to your pituitary. Courier hormones from your pituitary are then sent through your bloodstream to your adrenal cortex, prompting the release of hormones that speed up or slow down metabolic rates of cells through your body. Think of the adrenal cortex as a radio station broadcasting hormone signals to tissues, and the pituitary as the network hub that first sends the program (via a satellite link) to the affiliate station. Your hypothalamus—where the instructions originate—is like the production studio at the hub station.

Your adrenal cortex manufactures other hormones from progesterone in addition to the sex-related hormones. Among these are two very important steroid hormones, *cortisol* and *aldosterone*.

Cortisol is the scientific term for the more familiar *cortisone*, one of the first adrenal steroids isolated and used medically. In large quantities it reduces inflammation and suppresses certain immune responses. (Now we understand the success stories we're hearing about arthritis pains subsiding with the use of natural progesterone cream.)

Cortisol's primary function is to maintain adequate blood sugar levels by supporting faster glucose output when needed (an energy source), thereby helping you to cope with stress—emotional or physical.

Cortisol also contributes to the regulation of the day/night activity cycles.

Aldosterone is the hormone that controls potassium excretion and sodium retention—designed to accommodate a time long past when diets had an abundance of potassium and a shortage of sodium. Natural foods contain more potassium than sodium, but today, because 80 percent of our foods are processed, these metabolic functions appear to be contrary to need. The typical North American diet consists of far more sodium than potassium, throwing an important health-promoting ratio askew. You might be better served if your hormones and organs were more efficient at *retaining potassium* and *removing sodium*![3] Aldosterone is suppressed in the presence of potassium deficiency (or more typically, sodium excess).[4] Note the difference in the sodium and potassium ratios between processed and unprocessed foods in Table 1 on the next page.

Aldosterone also affects fluid retention and blood pressure, partly to help keep sodium and potassium in balance. So progesterone deficiency can result in aldosterone imbalance, leading to bloat, water retention, and blood pressure abnormalities.

You can see how varied and sensitive hormone secretion can be in response to environment, and how the presence of progesterone—the primary hormone responsible for cortisol and aldosterone production—has so many far-reaching physical effects. *Note that synthetic estrogen is a major contributor to progesterone deficiency!*

TABLE 1
POTASSIUM & SODIUM CONTENT
OF INTACT & PROCESSED FOODS
in milligrams/100 grams food
(100 grams is approximately 3½ oz, or the amount of food equal to the size of a closed fist)

	Potassium	Sodium
Flour, whole	360	3
White bread	100	540
Pork, uncooked	270	065
Bacon, uncooked	250	1400
Beef, uncooked	280	55
Corned beef	140	950
Haddock, uncooked	300	120
Haddock, smoked	190	790
Cabbage, uncooked	390	7
Cabbage, boiled	130	230
Horseradish, raw	564	8
Horseradish, prepared	290	96
Asparagus, raw	310	2
Asparagus, canned	250	200
Peas, fresh	380	1
Peas, frozen	135	125
Peas, canned	096	236
Peas, canned, served with ½ oz salted butter	099	374

Reprinted from *Everything You Always Wanted to Know About Potassium, But Were Too Tired To Ask*, Betty Kamen, Nutrition Encounter, 1992

Androgen is the third and, for us, the most interesting output of the adrenal cortex. *Dehydroepiandrosterone*, or DHEA (you can see why it is referred to by its initials), is the principal androgen made in the adrenals. Both testosterone and estradiol can be made from DHEA (recall that estradiol is an estrogen). In fact, before puberty DHEA is the major raw material for these hormones. This is important because testosterone and estradiol also have roles as growth hormones. DHEA is converted to stronger androgens, like testosterone, or to estradiol, as required.

> **Normalizing progesterone levels increases your natural production of DHEA.**

No testosterone is used by the brain—it's all made into an estrogen first. Keep this in mind if a male ever accuses you of not being able to "think like a man"!

At puberty, the male testes take over androgen production, surpassing the amount produced by the adrenal cortex. This corresponds to the adolescent growth spurt in boys, when skeletal muscles suddenly grow at a much greater rate under the influence of this new supply of male/growth hormones. The testes continue to produce androgens for life. Women, however, must rely on the adrenal cortex for androgenic hormones. Why do women need androgens? Primarily because of their tissue-building activity.

Estrogens and progesterone are produced by the ovaries between puberty and menopause. After menopause, the adrenal cortex is called on again to maintain what we once thought was the only supply of these vital hormones at this stage. We now know that ovaries can still produce a good supply of estrogen, even after menopause (as do fat cells and other body cells, too!).

Bursts of activity from your hypothalamus and pituitary attempt to restimulate your ovaries into maintaining estrogen levels at this time, and may even succeed. *These surges of control hormones are one source of hot flashes.* Your pituitary gland also has a role in controlling metabolism and body temperature—part of the reason for the "hot" in the hot flash.

What about progesterone? Figure 5 on page 42 shows the process (greatly simplified) by which your adrenal cortex manufactures steroid hormones. Starting with cholesterol (which can be stored to some extent in your adrenal gland, but should also be well supplied by your bloodstream), the first step is conversion to a substance called *pregnenolone*. Pregnenolone production normally controls the rate at which *all* the other steroid hormones can be created.[5]

The next maneuver is the construction of either progesterone or DHEA. Through a number of progressions not shown, the end result is any one of a series of hormones.

Many physicians warn about taking DHEA in supplemental form. They administer this hormone under strict medical surveillance, a determination made by tests and history. DHEA can make a big difference for those for whom it is indicated. It may enter either the estrogen or androgen pathways (Figure 5 on page 42), influenced by diet, genetics, overall health, and liver function. If you have had endometriosis, breast cancer, uterine pain (caused by estrogen excess), or you are overweight (in which case you may have excess estrogen because of surplus fatty tissue), supplemental DHEA is not for you, as it may increase your estrogen "load."

Dr. Corsello points out that endocrinology, in addition to being a science, is also an art. (See page 252 for more information on DHEA.)

FIGURE 5

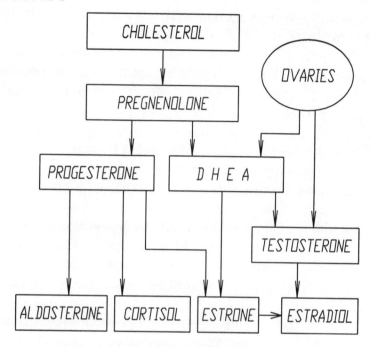

PATHWAYS FROM CHOLESTEROL
TO SEX HORMONES

This shows the chemical pathway from cholesterol to some important sex hormones that are synthesized in the adrenal cortex (simplified). Notice that there are several ways to make the estrogens *estrone* and *estradiol*.

A national news announcement informed Americans that progestins can thin vaginal walls, thereby increasing susceptibility to the HIV virus. Again: progesterone infers that the hormone is natural; progistin, that it is synthetic. Synthetic progestins were used in this study, not the natural hormone!

There's something very significant about the pathways shown in Figure 5. As noted, there are two possible chemical routes to get to the estrogens. One involves progesterone as the main intermediate step, while the other route bypasses progesterone and uses DHEA. So while progesterone is an important hormonal building block for estrogen production, it can be used to a greater or lesser extent for this purpose, depending on how much is available. It's like going from one city to another using an interstate highway or getting there by traveling the back roads. You use a different route, but end up in the same place.

Progesterone is also manufactured in massive quantities by the placenta during pregnancy. The accelerated production starts in the fourth month and can reach 300 or more milligrams a day. This is 10 to 15 times the amount produced by your ovaries before pregnancy! If you have given birth to a child, you may remember the freedom from headaches and general feeling of well-being—even euphoria—that you felt as you began to enter your second trimester. High progesterone levels during pregnancy are believed to be responsible for the exhilaration.[6]

Progesterone levels vary with the menstrual cycle, and its deficiency is considered to be closely linked to mood swings associated with PMS. Estrogen excess during the second half of the cycle is the problem. Estrogen and progesterone are in competition with each other at some receptor sites. In the presence of enough progesterone, estrogen is displaced, cancelling many of the effects caused by too much estrogen. If progesterone levels are low, however, estrogen dominates. Even if both progesterone and estrogen are low, estrogen will be elevated.[7] And herein lies the trouble.

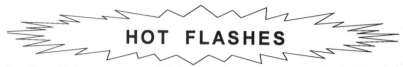

HOT FLASHES

➤ Synthetic progestins and natural progesterone have only one common function: ability to sustain secretory endometrium. Progestins don't have the full spectrum of progesterone's activity.

Clinical Use of Sex Steroids, 1980[8]

➤ Progestins have an adverse effect on insulin resistance. They can also raise triglycerides, and are related to breast cancer risk.

American Jnl of Obstetrics & Gynecology, 1994[9]
Monographs/National Cancer Institute, 1994[10]

➤ Synthetic progestins have a wide variety of side effects.

Clinical Use of Sex Steroids, 1980[11]

➤ Natural progesterone shows improved lipid profile, amenorrhea without endometrial problems, and has no side effects.

Optimal Health Guidelines, 1992[12]

➤ Any change in the molecular configuration of steroids alters their effects.

Optimal Health Guidelines, 1992[13]

➤ Natural progesterone is an attractive means of supplementation in postmenopausal HRT without any liver-related side effects.

Gynecological Endocrinology, 1993[14]

UPDATES

Lancet 1997 Feb 15;349(9050):458-61
Postmenopausal women who use combined therapy of estrogen with cyclic progestagen have an increased risk of endometrial cancer, even when progestagen is added for 10 or more days per month.

International Journal of Cancer 1996 Jul 29;67:327-32
Exposure to an estrogen-progestin combined brand is associated with increased risk of breast cancer.

~~ **ENDNOTES** ~~ *The fantasy continues...*

We know we'll say good-bye to menstruation some day. Perhaps we already have.

There are unpleasant memories, like the day of overflow when we wore our white skirt or white pants. There are pleasant memories, like the time we did or didn't want to be pregnant and our period did or didn't appear.

It's hard to imagine societies, even primitive ones, that did not have the use of mini- or maxi-pads.

Whatever our *external* practices to catch the menstrual rivulet, very few of us really know the *inside* story. So, back we go into ourselves in our fantasy, to watch in awe as estrogen and progesterone and other hormones fluctuate up and down, vying with each other for supremacy here, working in tandem there.

Ah! And now we see exactly why the chocolate cake we had for dinner interferes with the natural course of some of these events, and why PMS takes hold more readily in the presence of such indiscretions.

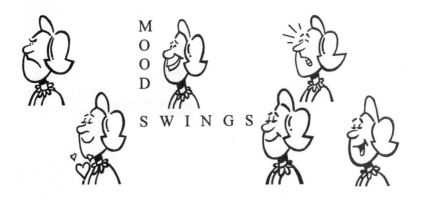

MOOD SWINGS

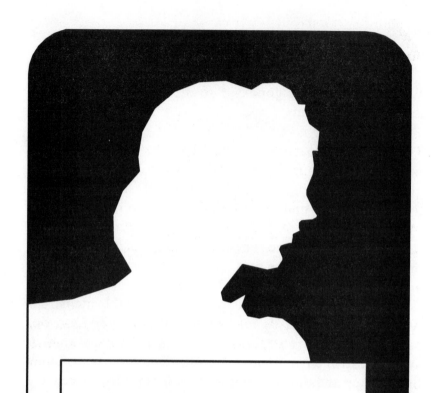

4

HORMONES AND
THE MENSTRUAL CYCLE

FRIEND OR FOE?

My friend Susan speaks for many women when she says, "Menstruation makes me feel integrated, body and mind. It reminds me that I am *all* that I am—that what I think and feel and want has much to do with what is going on with me hormonally, nutritionally, and biochemically. It reminds me of this in a good way. When I get a little PMS, or a little crampy, I take it as a message that there's something imbalanced that needs my attention."[1]

Times have changed! When I was a teenager, menstruation was a word to be uttered in whispers. If you told your best friend that you "fell off the roof" (and you *only* told your best friend), she knew that you were menstruating.

Menstruation was known as "the poorlies" in nineteenth century America, "the curse" in the twentieth century, and in France you can still hear, "I'm going to see Sophie." But the very oldest word for menstruation means "the woman's friend."

Beth Richards, in *Blood of the Moon*, comments: "The simple fact that menstruation has evolved from 'woman's friend' to 'the curse' is a powerful symbol of the status of women."[2]

It may also be indicative of our declining health.

As recently as 1970, Dr. Edgar Berman had PMS in mind when he declared that women weren't suitable for leadership positions because of their "raging hormonal influences." And as currently as 1993, the American Psychiatric Association concluded that women with severe PMS actually have a psychiatric disorder. In their current manual, PMS is cited under "mental disorders—not otherwise specified." If this arches your back, hear more: This group now wants to label the condition *"premenstrual dysphoric disorder"* (PMDD), a specifically-defined psychiatric derangement under mood and depression.

How do you feel about a category of mental disorder that includes only women? *Newsweek* comments about this citation: "Chances are there will be tears, irrationality and outbursts of anger— *elicited by neither hormones nor mental illness*."[3]

Even worse: In 1994 an article in *American Journal for Clinical Nutrition* was headlined "Premenstrual syndrome does exist!" This journal is published for physicians. Do physicians have to be convinced, even now? The *Obstetrical and Gynecological Survey* stated that "PMS is probably a group of entities which includes various symptoms that occur during the 7 to 10 days before menstruation and disappears a few hours after the onset of menstruation." *Probably*? Aren't we nearing the end of the twentieth century? Where have these researchers/physicians been?

UNDERSTANDING MENSTRUATION

While women seek therapeutic help for PMS, lack of understanding of its etiology causes treatment to be focused on symptoms rather than underlying initiating factors. The result of constructive advice for this poorly understood problem has often been the administration of drugs. But a risk-benefit appraisal, published in *Drug Safety,* reveals that adverse effects of these medications outweigh their benefits. *Let's find out what really goes on.*

Figure 6 on page 50 shows the levels of estrogen and progesterone over a typical 28-day menstrual cycle. It also indicates a few of the control hormones produced by your pituitary.[4] In your effort to make decisions about hormone therapy, you may find it extremely beneficial to spend a few minutes with this chart.

Note that Day 1 represents the day that menstrual flow begins, and that ovulation occurs at Day 14, stimulated by hormones. The 28-day cycle is average. A cycle that varies in both length and time of ovulation may not be abnormal— anything from a 20- to 40-day cycle may be okay. What's not okay is the presence of PMS. Women with irregular cycles and/or extended days of heavy flow, however, can dramatically turn things around after positive alterations in diet and lifestyle—especially with the *right* kind of HRT!

We'll start our narrative on Day 5 or so, when the menstrual flow subsides. This is the beginning of the pre-ovulatory, or *follicular* phase of the cycle, named for the follicles (the containers for the ovum, or eggs) in your ovaries.

FIGURE 6

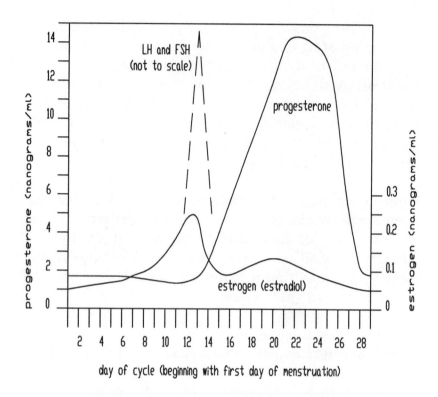

TYPICAL PROGESTERONE
AND ESTROGEN LEVELS
DURING THE 28-DAY CYCLE

Note that concentrations of the two hormones are plotted on different scales. Where curves cross, 20 times more progesterone than estrogen circulates in the bloodstream.

Concentrations of progesterone and estrogen (estradiol) vary over the 28-day menstrual cycle. When progesterone peaks, there should be about 140 times as much progesterone as estrogen.

FIGURE 7

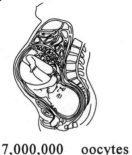

7,000,000 oocytes

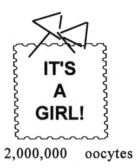

2,000,000 oocytes

400,000 oocytes

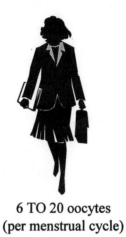

6 TO 20 oocytes
(per menstrual cycle)

FOLLICLE REDUCTION RATE

When you reach puberty, each ovary contains about 400,000 follicles, down-sized from about 7,000,000 after six months of embryonic life, and about 2,000,000 at birth. Each of these follicles contains an *oocyte.* (Each "o" is pronounced separately, so it's o-o-cyte.) An oocyte is the human egg cell, the largest of all human cells. But only six to twenty of these begin to develop during a menstrual cycle, and only one continues to develop in only one ovary!

FIGURE 8

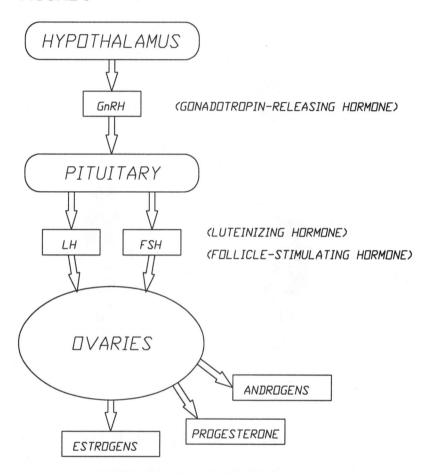

LINKS BETWEEN THE BRAIN AND
SEX HORMONE PRODUCTION

Chemical links between your brain and sex hormone production are complex. Your hypothalamus is partially controlled by nerve signals. It sends chemical messages to your pituitary, which produces hormones through intricate pathways. In turn, these hormones stimulate your ovaries to go through various phases of ovulation and hormone production.

Development of the egg cell is sparked by the brain-controlled hypothalamus through a hormone called *gonado-tropin-releasing hormone*, or GnRH. GnRH stimulates your pituitary to release two more substances into your bloodstream: *luteinizing hormone* (LH) and *follicle-stimulating hormone* (FSH). These in turn act directly on your ovaries where they promote:

(1) Development and enlargement of follicles
(2) The production of estrogen by the follicle cells
   (See Figure 8 on page 52.)

The estrogen produced this way has an interesting effect. *It makes the follicles generate even more estrogen.* This is called a positive feedback loop. It's something like holding a microphone too close to a loudspeaker. Sound comes out of the speaker, the sound is picked up by the microphone, gets amplified, and comes out of the speaker much louder—where it gets picked up again by the microphone. The result is an ear-splitting electronic whistle that doesn't go away until the volume is turned down or the microphone is turned off or covered.

Hormone interactions during the follicular phase of the menstrual cycle work in essentially the same way, but they have the added complication of a *multiple* feedback loop. (See Figure 9 on page 54.) The estrogen made by your ovaries surrounding the follicles tends to increase production in at least three different ways:

(1) By stimulating your hypothalamus to produce more GnRH, which, in turn, stimulates your pituitary and ovaries
(2) By stimulating your pituitary to make more LH and FSH, which stimulates your ovaries
(3) By increasing the sensitivity of the cells surrounding the follicles in your ovaries to respond even *more* to the LH and FSH from your pituitary

FIGURE 9

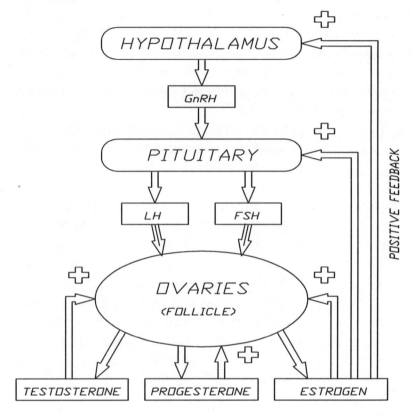

FOLLICULAR PHASE OF THE MENSTRUAL CYCLE BETWEEN MENSTRUATION AND OVULATION

Hormones produced by the ovarian follicles have a positive feedback effect. More estrogen stimulates the hypothalamus to make more GnRH, causing the pituitary to make more LH and FSH, which stimulates the ovarian follicles to produce even more estrogen. The plus signs indicate the positive feedback loop, activating glands to produce more hormones. Higher estrogen concentration leads to *more* estrogen production.

Follicles also communicate chemically with each other through a mechanism not yet fully understood. Only one follicle in one ovary continues to develop throughout the cycle. The egg-producing ovary sends a message to the other ovary to refrain from doing the same. *The presence of progesterone initiates this "cease and desist" order.* The growth of the chosen follicle continues to accelerate. During the last two days before ovulation this follicle may be as large as 20 millimeters in diameter—over three-quarters of an inch!

FIGURE 10

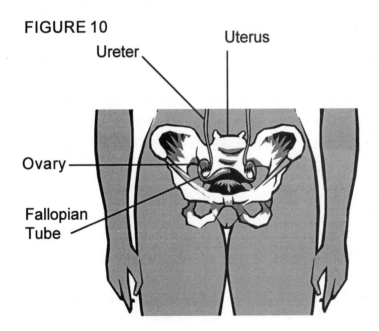

FEMALE REPRODUCTIVE SYSTEM

The ovary is 1¼ inches long. The uterus is a hollow muscular organ 3 inches in length. The Fallopian tube is a 4½-inch tunnel to the uterus.

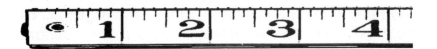

Progesterone is also responsible for increased female libido. This makes sense because of its associated production at the time of maximum fertility.

In a certain island culture where yams containing progesterone-like substances are a major staple of the diet, libido is high but birth rate is low. The ample supply of these substances during the first half of the menstrual cycle may be responsible for reducing the rate of ovulation, while sex drive remains high throughout the month. (These people appear to be *extremely* happy!)

The amount of yam extract in cream preparations is not high enough to have this contraceptive effect, but it appears to be high enough to normalize libido.

Back to business. On Day 14 of the cycle, LH and FSH swell to high levels, and this is known as the *pre-ovulatory surge*. The follicle moves to the wall of the ovary, enzymes degrade the ovary wall at the site of the protrusion, and the ovum is ejected from the follicle into your abdominal cavity. From there it finds its way to one of your Fallopian tubes for slow transportation to your uterus (and possible fertilization by a sperm on the way).

Don't think the follicle is done with its work. Immediately after release of the ovum on Day 14, the remaining cells continue to function. The follicle is now called the *corpus luteum*, and the post-ovulatory phase is called the *luteal phase* of the menstrual cycle. The corpus luteum is rich in cholesterol, conferring both its yellow color and its name. The word *luteal* means yellow.

FIGURE 11

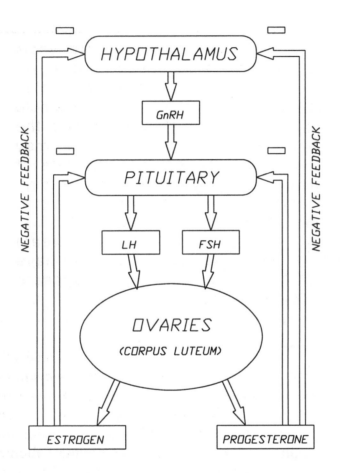

EVENTS FOLLOWING OVULATION

During the luteal phase, the feedback becomes negative. Estrogen and especially progesterone now inhibit the hypothalamus and pituitary from stimulating the ovaries into producing more hormones. The minus signs indicate suppression of glandular hormone production.

The follicle continues to produce estrogen, *but it also begins to manufacture a large amount of progesterone.* This grand flow of progesterone helps to suppress the development of other follicles so that only one follicle ejects an ovum. If, by chance, both of the ovaries have follicles that eject an ovum at almost exactly the same time — which happens about once every 300 periods—the result can be fraternal twins.

What about the runaway feedback loop? High levels of progesterone come to the rescue, shutting off the lofty rate of production of estrogen, GnRH, LH, and FSH. (See Figure 11 on page 57.) Circulating progesterone has an inhibiting effect on the production of GnRH by your hypothalamus and on the production of LH and FSH by your pituitary. The corpus luteum remains in your ovary and continues to grow for seven or eight days following ovulation. Then it degenerates, at which time progesterone and estrogen return to their initial levels.

During the luteal phase after ovulation, estrogen and progesterone stimulate growth and proliferation of the blood vessels and connective tissue in the wall of the uterus, ready to provide support and nutrients if a fertilized ovum is implanted.

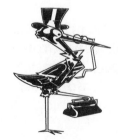

"With natural progesterone supplements, pregnancies which went to term were significantly better, resulting in a 94 percent success rate."
Jnl Gynecol Obstet Biol Reprod, 1993;22:471-5

If fertilization hasn't occurred about eight days after ovulation, this growth reverses, and your menstrual phase begins. *Prostaglandins* (those produced by your uterus) stimulate muscles within uterine walls, making them contract rhythmically and expel all the blood-rich and degenerating connective tissue from the inner surface of your uterine wall.

Throughout this process, the balance between estrogen and progesterone is critical. Progesterone is a good anti-spasmodic. Low progesterone levels will affect not only your uterus, but smooth muscles in general, so it is cramp- and migraine-related. (See page 212 for hints for relieving PMS cramps and migraines.) Maintaining an adequate level of progesterone is particularly important—especially during the luteal phase when progesterone is keeping the positive feedback loop in check. *The prostaglandins that contract your uterus can also cause contractions in other involuntary muscles. This is what causes menstrual cramps and PMS migraines.*

You can see how evidence is beginning to point to a certain strategy for dealing with PMS. Maintaining your ability to produce progesterone and avoiding external sources of estrogen wherever possible are critical measures. External sources of estrogen come from beef, chickens, eggs, dairy products loaded with hormones (both from the animals' feed and from implantation in animals), and from foreign estrogens emitted into our environment from herbicides, pesticides, industrial pollution, and plastics. (See page 251.)

I believe that when progesterone and estrogen are in proper balance for everyone, premenstrual syndrome will be nothing more than words in an outdated medical book.

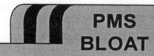

MEMOS

PMS BLOAT

A Few Facts About PMS and Bloat

➢ Of course one should *never* drive and drink, but least of all just before your period! That's when you will show higher blood levels of alcohol. Premenstrual bloating probably accounts for this, since alcohol levels parallel those of body water. The lowest levels occur on the first day of menstrual bleeding.

➢ To reduce premenstrual bloating:
~ Balance sodium/potassium intake. Additional information on how to do this is available in my book, *Everything You Always Wanted to Know About Potassium But Were Too Tired to Ask.*[5]

~ Add natural progesterone to your daily regimen. (See suggestions later in this book.)

~ Don't use Stimerol chewing gum. It contains glycyrrhizinic acid, a main component of licorice, which can induce sodium retention.[6]

~ Use large amounts of acidophilus, both orally and vaginally. The presence of yeast can cause bloating, but a good supply of friendly bacteria helps to solve the problem.

~ Wheat sensitivity, a problem more prevalent than generally recognized, can contribute to bloat. Try eliminating wheat products for one month to see what happens. My guess is you'll be pleasantly surprised.

MEMOS 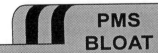 **PMS BLOAT**

➢ The increased levels of sex steroids occurring during a normal menstrual cycle affect caffeine elimination. Clearance of caffeine is slower in the luteal phase.[7] Caffeine disturbs pH, which contributes to PMS.

➢ Vascular congestion may lead to water retention. Sexual activity relieves such congestion.[8]

➢ Natural herbal diuretics include raspberry leaf, marjoram, and thyme teas, available at health stores. These herbs do not have the damaging effects of prescription diuretics.[9]

➢ Vitamin B_6 is especially valuable in reducing premenstrual edema.[10] (Whenever you consume a single faction of the B complex, be sure to add a product containing the *whole* of the B complex. Examples: Green kamut concentrate, chlorella, bee pollen, brewer's yeast.)

➢ Drugs that function as diuretics can have serious side effects. They require close medical supervision with regular blood tests to check body salt balance. Overuse of diuretics can upset potassium and sodium levels, which can make PMS worse.[11]

➢ Common symptoms are shared by women complaining of PMS and menopause.

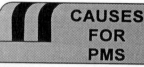

MEMOS

CAUSES FOR PMS

➢ Possible causes for PMS:
  ~ progesterone deficiency
  ~ estrogen/progesterone imbalance
  ~ thyroid hypofunction
  ~ antidiuretic hormone excess
  ~ fluid retention
  ~ shifting endorphin levels
  ~ serotonin alterations
  ~ abnormal prostaglandin action
  ~ vitamin deficiency (especially B_6)
  ~ ovarian infection
  ~ yeast overgrowth
  ~ hypoglycemia
  ~ neuroendocrine disorders
  ~ abnormal blood pressure and
    heart rates
  ~ abnormal renal handling of water
  ~ opioid dysfunction
  ~ reduced magnesium levels
  ~ vitamin D deficiency
  ~ zinc deficiency (and copper excess)

French Journal, 1995[12]
Psychosomatic Medicine, 1994[13]
Journal of Affective Disorders, 1994[14]
*Journal of Clinical Endocrinology &
    Metabolism,* 1993[15]
Obstetrics & Gynecology, 1994[16]
Fertility & Sterility, 1994[17]
Journal of Reproductive Medicine, 1993[18]
Gynecologica Scandinavica, 1994[19]

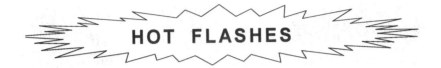

HOT FLASHES

➤ Although depression may be a symptom of PMS, depressive disorders do not *cause* PMS.
> *Psychosomatices, 1995*[20]
> *Psychosomatic Medicine, 1994*[21]

➤ Lack of ovulation is common for intensive athletes who do not supplement. It is also common in those who limit food intake excessively without supplementation.
> *Pediatric Clinics of North America, 1989*[22]

➤ Food choices are often responsive to the hormonal changes in your menstrual cycle.
> *American Jnl of Clinical Nutrition, 1993*[23]

➤ Consumption of foods and beverages high in sugar is associated with the prevalence of PMS.
> *Jnl of Reproductive Medicine, 1991*[24]

➤ Women with PMS might have disturbances of their hypothalamus and adrenal glands.
> *Jnl of Clin Endocrinology & Metabolism, 1990*[25]

➤ Supplemental tryptophan reduced the following symptoms of PMS: irritability, insomnia, and carbohydrate craving.
> *Jnl of Psychiatry & Neuroscience, 1994*[26]

➤ Free radicals (highly reactive particles caused by toxins or rancidity, as found in salad dressings and other processed foods) play a role in the regression of the corpus luteum.
> *Jnl of Reproduction and Fertility, 1992*[27]

➤ Menstrual problems which include amenorrhea (lack of menstruation), irregular cycles, or abnormal uterine bleeding represent 50 percent of adolescent gynecologic complaints. Amenorrhea may also be a sign of late puberty or of a problem affecting the hypothalamus, the pituitary, or the ovaries.
> *Hormone Research, 1991*[28]

UPDATES

Jnl of Psychosomatic Obstet Gynaecol 1996 Mar;17:21
Women diagnosed as having PMS do not respond in a uniform fashion to ovarian hormones.

Delaware Medical Jnl 1996 Jul;68(7):357-63
Many physicians [still] do not believe that PMS exists. Special interest groups also dispute its existence.

1996 Medical Tribune News Service
Water helps to increase urine volume, which in turn helps flush bacteria from the bladder. Cranberry pills are more effective than cranberry juice. Restricting the amount of acid can intensify bladder inflammation.

Archives of Family Medicine 1996;5:593-596
Vaginal infections can be warded off by consuming yogurt or taking dietary supplements that contain a live bacteria known as lactobacillus acidophilus.

1996 *Amer Col of Obst and Gyn Report*
Pain is caused when hormones causing your uterine lining to thicken and shed each month during your period has a similar effect on the tissue growing outside your uterus. Tissue bleeds and sheds, and may form painful cysts and lesions.

Psychosomatic Medicine 1995 Jul-Aug;57(4):324-30
[Processed] carbohydrate consumption and eating behavior are associated with menstrual distress.

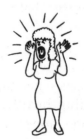

"Mom is yelling again.
It must be that time of month."

"I need some chocolate.
It must be that time of month."

IT DOESN'T HAVE TO BE THIS WAY!

~~ ENDNOTES ~~ *The fantasy continues...*

Aging, and the decades move on. We note how much more slowly repair cells make their way toward a scratch, how diminished in number they are for the mending, how much longer it takes for replacement cells to reach suntanned skin. The bountiful supply of organ reserve abates—a nest egg granted with such generosity to youth.

See the negative effects of toxins—in constant battle with immune cells. See the benefits of antioxidants—hopefully, the victors. Watch as mushed and mangled foods produce warriors—fighting the wrong cause. Watch the nutrient-dense foods as they provide ammunition for triumph. Note that more of the good guys are required today than yesterday—because we are one day older.

Can we learn from experience? Will we acknowledge today that we need more of the support system tomorrow because we will have aged yet another 24 hours?

Aging—it takes us by surprise. Our ovaries put up a sign: *Going Out of Business.* Nature seems to be saying, "We don't need any more like you." *Not to worry:* nature doesn't want us to go without. *Another organ gets pressed into service.* Nor do the ovaries totally close their doors!

We observe that wrinkling occurs more rapidly in one woman than another. The fantasy demonstrates exactly *how* and *why* aging changes take place at menopause. We note that a menopausal woman *can* continue to manufacture hormones—just the right amount to maintain optimal health, including healthy bones and a healthy sex life. But the message appears to be:
   Now we need a little more help.

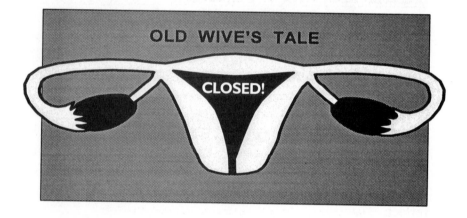

5

HORMONES AND MENOPAUSE

IT DOESN'T HAVE TO BE BAD NEWS

Happy 50th birthday! If you are an average American woman celebrating a half century of life, chances are your varicose veins and your tummy stick out, your dimples and breasts sag, and the mirror reveals a bigger nose and droopier earlobes than ever before. (Too bad those glasses make your vision so perfect.) Your doctor, however, is concerned about a change that your mirror does not directly reflect: *The slowdown of hormone production!*

Happy birthday? Actually, the processes leading to these aging overtures began decades before this landmark year. Various parts of your skeleton, for example, started their downslide when you were in your twenties. You can be sure there has been a constant reduction of the mechanical properties of your bone with age—even if tests which your physician may have administered show no loss of bone density until you approach menopause.[1] (An inexpensive test using *photons*, which are beams of very high intensity light, can now define the status of your bone density with great accuracy.)

The output of very important hormones start their plunge in your thirties. In fact, in some ways you begin to age from the moment you are born.

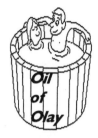

You can bathe in Oil of Olay forever, but you will get old—if that is all you use in your attempt to delay the visual impact of the aging process!

The news, however, is not totally negative. As Hallmark cards inform us, *Fifty Can Be Nifty!* Adrenal glands pump estrogens even as ovaries slow their manufacture. Although adrenal estrogen is not as powerful as ovarian estrogen, your body is most appreciative for the offering. Called *estrone*, this contribution is converted from weak male hormones in fat cells. The healthier your adrenals, the less apt you are to suffer common menopausal complaints— depression, sweating, vaginal dryness, loss of libido, and that devilish dynamic duo, *hot flashes and wakeful nights.*

Significantly more fatty tissue is concentrated just below the abdominal skin of perimenopausal women (the years prior to menopause).[2] The tendency for women to experience "middle-age spread" may not be without purpose or benefit. Heavier women have the least severe osteoporotic symptoms. Don't get too excited about the benefits of overweight, however: *Estrogenic hormone levels are usually more out of balance in those who are overweight, especially in the presence of progesterone deficiency.*

Menstrual cycles often become irregular as you approach menopause. Even when you do menstruate, you may not ovulate—despite normal estrogen levels.

> Without the cyclic increase and fall in progesterone during the perimenopausal stage, endometrial shedding is not triggered in a timely fashion. So menstrual cycles become irregular.

Carpal tunnel syndrome is one disorder which tends to increase with menopause, resulting in pain and burning or tingling in the fingers and hand, sometimes extending to the elbow. Caused by the compression of a nerve, it has been known for more than a decade that carpal tunnel syndrome is linked to vitamin B_6 (pyridoxine) deficiency.[3] Vitamin B_6 in supplemental form, therefore, may be helpful. According to a report published in the *Annals of the New York Academy of Sciences*, 1990, vitamin B_6 is safe at doses of 100 milligrams a day.[4] The addition of a daily dose of magnesium (400 milligrams) along with the vitamin B_6 (50 milligrams) increases the benefit. It could take about 2 to 12 weeks for this remedy to work. Although carpal tunnel syndrome is common among both male and female computer keyboard users, hormonal changes at menopause appear to exacerbate the condition for women.[5]

Now let's dispel a few menopause myths.

> Within a month, one journal reported that menopause is primarily represented as a medical condition, while another described menopause as "not a disease."
>
> *Primary Care*
> 1997 Mar;24(1):205-21
> *American Jnl of Preventive Medicine*
> 1997 Jan-Feb;13:58

WHAT MENOPAUSE WON'T DO

➤ Menopause itself does not cause significant weight gain. No serious differences are found between pre- and postmenopausal women with regard to total body weight, body mass index, waist-hip ratio, and *total* abdominal fat tissue areas.

International Journal of Obesity, 1992[6]

➤ Popular medical view to the contrary, natural menopause does not have negative mental health consequences for middle-aged healthy women.

Journal of Consulting & Clinical Psychology, 1990[7]

WHAT MENOPAUSE WILL DO

➤ Blood pressure increases with age—or, more accurately, as a result of aging in people living the usual Western lifestyle with its destructive dietary habits. *Ovarian failure appears to be protective against this increase.*

American Journal of Epidemiology, 1989[8]

➤ Estradiol, a form of estrogen, enhances vulnerability to schizophrenia, but the effect is lowered during menopause.

European Archives of Psychiatry and Clinical Neuroscience, 1991[9]

➤ Menopause brings with it a total freedom from pregnancy concern, and, for many, a new level of sexual enjoyment because of this freedom.

Healthy menopausal women the world over

MISCELLANEOUS MENOPAUSE FACTS

➤ A woman in the United States can now expect to live for thirty years or more past menopause.
Drug Intelligence and Clinical Pharmacy, 1988[10]

➤ The earlier the menopause, the greater the need to improve lifestyle or seek the right kind of treatment.
Union Medicale du Canada, 1992[11]

➤ Bone loss related to menopause begins during the irregular menstruation period *before* menopause.
Calcified Tissue International, 1991[12]

➤ Regular sexual activity is beneficial in maintaining a healthy, functional vagina.
Postgraduate Medicine, 1992[13]

➤ High intake of dietary fiber, vitamin C, and beta-carotene decrease the risk for postmenopausal breast cancer.
International Journal of Cancer, 1991[14]

➤ The time between menopause and the occurrence of hip fractures averages about 30 years. [Some physicians place this number at 10 or 15 years.]
Lancet, 1993[15]

➤ Osteoporosis begins several years prior to menopause, *before any decrease in estrogen levels.*
Canadian Journal of Obstetrics and Gynecology, 1991[16]

Note this last fact: *Osteoporosis begins several years before menopause, yet estrogen levels are normal up to the time of menopause.* More about this later!

AGE AT MENOPAUSE

At the turn of the century, the average menopausal woman in this country was about 45. Today, the average age of the *climactic*, as it is called in the medical literature, is closer to 50 or 51.

For reasons not understood, age at menopause is significantly earlier among left-handed women than those who are right-handed.[17]

Active smokers experience menopause 1.7 years sooner than non-smokers. The typical age of onset in nonsmokers is 49.8; in passive smokers (nonsmokers who live or work with smokers), it's 49.1; and in active smokers, it's 48.13 years. These differences depend on the duration of smoking— increasing with the number of smoked cigarettes to as much as 2.4 years earlier in smokers of more than 20 cigarettes per day, and to 3 years earlier if your mother was also a smoker.[18]

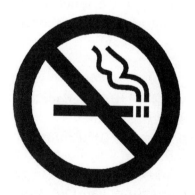

Evidence suggests that cigarette smoking has an anti-estrogenic effect in women.[19]

HOT FLASHES

A group of investigators examined Japanese women among whom hot flashes are infrequent. They found a high intake of both *phytoestrogens* (100- to 1,000-fold more than in American women) and other foods which have estrogen activity.[20] This represents an example of how plant foods can modulate your hormone metabolism.

Phytoestrogen foods contain a group of substances called *isoflavones*, which are weak estrogen-like constituents that act as *adaptogens*. If a woman has an excessive amount of estrogen, these substances help to block the estrogen from entering estrogen receptor sites. If there is not enough estrogen, they fill the gap. An interesting study published in the *Journal of the National Cancer Institute* (1994;86:174) explains this adaptogenic phenomenon. The estrogenic activity of phytoestrogens is one reason why hot flashes are not as common among Japanese women.

Phytoestrogens are associated with soy products (tofu, miso, aburage, atuage, koridofu, soybeans, boiled soy beans, and sprouted soy beans). Tofu offers the most phytoestrogenic activity of the soy-based foods, and soy milk the least. Other phytoestrogen-containing foods are black cohosh, alfalfa, licorice, and pomegranates.

But don't get too excited about adding soy products to your diet, unless you have a good, organic source. Soybeans are genetically engineered by one of our top producers to withstand high doses of the herbicide "Roundup," a crop weed killer. These genetically engineered soy products have never been tested on humans. We know that allergens can be transferred through genetic engineering, and that most herbicides of this type are contaminated with a suspected carcinogen. It is no wonder that more than 100 European retailers, food manufacturers, and food processors have refused to accept our genetically engineered soybeans. (This news makes the case for natural progesterone supplementation essential, as explained later.)

Women have reported that they have fewer and less intense hot flashes when they have a fever. The reasons? Perhaps the following:

(1) Because of competing heat-regulatory drives, the characteristic changes do not occur. The temperature inhibits whatever it is that launches the hot flash.

(2) Some product of the fever process masks the changes that occur during hot flashes.[21]

We don't need double-blind, randomly controlled studies to tell us that those who experience hot flashes during the night tend to sleep less efficiently. But it sure is hopeful to know that such information is cited in the medical literature, as in the journal, *Sleep.*[22] The professionals are finally paying attention.

Vitamin E has a stabilizing effect on estrogen levels, so supplementation with this fat-soluble nutrient may increase hormone production in those who are vitamin E-deficient. The increased hormone production caused by supplemental vitamin E helps to reduce hot flashes. Vitamin C and bioflavonoids have also been beneficial.

Many questions about hot flashes remain unanswered. According to the *New York Academy of Sciences,* the flashes may start much earlier and continue far longer than is commonly recognized by physicians or acknowledged in textbooks of gynecology. Hot flashes are not static; patterns may change with time. For some women, they become less frequent and less intense; for others, they may continue at hourly intervals well into old age.[23]

IT DOESN'T HAVE TO BE THIS WAY!

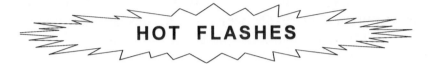

HOT FLASHES

➢ Women who smoke in the premenopausal stage and those reporting natural menopause before age 52 have increased probability of hot flashes.

Obstetrics and Gynecology, 1994[24]

➢ Only five percent of women receiving ERT said they had requested the therapy from their practitioner.

British Jnl of General Practice, 1991[25]

➢ Certain steroid hormones are found in lesser quantities in women who experience early, rather than late, menopause.

Jnl of the Medical Assoc of Thailand, 1992[26]

➢ Glucose and cholesterol values are significantly higher in postmenopausal women.

International Jnl of Obesity, 1992[27]

➢ Eighty percent of women on replacement therapy say they would have liked more information about menopause before its onset.

British Jnl of General Practice, 1991[28]

➢ The antidepressant effects of estrogen therapy were examined in a large group of women 50 years of age. Those using estrogen had higher average depressive symptoms than women who had never used estrogen.

Obstetrics and Gynecology, 1992, 80:30

UPDATES

Maturitas 1997 Mar;26(2):73-82

"Menopause" is a word of multiple meanings. Once the subject of taboo, it is now almost in danger of overexposure. The result is a new level of confusion and even exploitation in the minds of the health profession and the public alike.

New England Jnl of Medicine 1997 Jun 19;336:1769-75
Postmenopausal ERT increases the risk of breast cancer. Survival benefits diminish with longer use.

Lancet 1997 Feb 15;349(9050):458-61
Postmenopausal estrogen therapy is associated with an increased risk of endometrial cancer. Combined therapy of estrogen with cyclic progestin of a long-term basis has an increased risk of endometrial cancer compared with no use of hormone therapy, even when progestin is added for 10 or more days per month.

Jnl of American Assoc Gyneco Laparosc 1996 Nov;4:13
Endometrial polyps can appear in menopausal women receiving hormone therapy despite the presence of progestins to oppose the action of estrogens.

Cancer Jnl Clinic 1996 Nov-Dec;46(6):365-73
In patients with hormonally sensitive tumors, estrogen replacement therapy carries a risk of stimulating recurrent disease as well as contributing to an increased risk of other hormonally related cancers.

British Jnl of Obstetrics & Gynecology 1997 Feb;104:163
Contraindications of five currently available estrogen preparations include cardiovascular disease, diabetes, liver diseases, osteosclerosis, endometriosis, melanoma, and hormone-dependent tumors.

New England Journal of Medicine 1995;333:1357
Women on (synthetic) hormones that delay menopause have a higher risk of breast cancer.

New England Jnl of Medicine, 1997, June 19; 336:1821
The protective effect of hormones is lost five years after discontinuation of use. Extended exposure provides no additional benefit. There is a 43 percent increase in deaths from breast cancer among those who use hormones 10 or more years.

~~ ENDNOTES ~~ *The fantasy continues...*

No matter how young we feel, our physical appearance reflects the aging process—especially when our fantasy escorts us to the internal architecture of our bones, enabling us to see the *disequilibrium* between normal bone formation and bone loss. We watch as our skeleton is constantly "doing and undoing." We see its changing density. Not much happens to size or shape—only to *porosity*. A fast-moving panorama helps us to observe osteoporosis setting in—a wooden rod replacing one of steel—but only in those who are not optimally nourished.

In our fantasy, science is advanced enough to understand the dynamics. We see *how* bone changes as it heals, shapes, and grows. We catch the magic of *how* calcium gets incorporated, *how* cartilage hardens, *how* vitamin C affects collagen. We see one kind of cell looking for old bone to dissolve: *Pacman wiping out its victims.* We follow with awe as another kind of cell gives birth to new bone: *the miracle of creation.*

Even at age 90, we note that bone can mend in the presence of bone-building tools. Now we know that bone is not unchanging, but forever shifting. We see that making this happen is dependent on life choices. We note how different it is when the appropriate nutrients are present. *Bone loss may be a natural accompaniment of aging, but it need not have adverse implications.*

We look at an older woman, and, because this is fantasy, we watch the aging process in reverse—70, 60, 40, 20, 10, 3. Now we see larger eyes, shorter nose, smoother skin, fuller cheeks, and bones so rubbery and supple they do not break during any fall. Once upon a time, that was us!

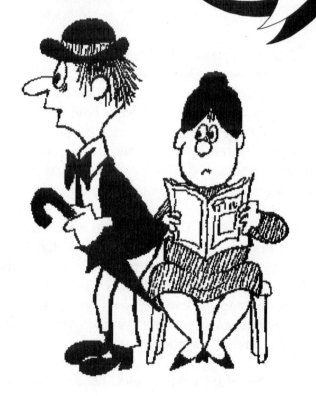

6

ABOUT BONE

BONE IS LIVING TISSUE

Bone is far more complicated than you might imagine. It's essentially a composite of two types of material: tendon-like organic collagen and hard inorganic calcium phosphate crystals. The combination can be likened to fiberglass, comprised of both flexible cloth and brittle plastic resin. Together, they make a consolidated structure that's strong and tough. Flexible, spongy collagen would be useless by itself as bone, just as the brittle calcium phosphate would fracture much too easily on its own. But they combine to make an amazingly enduring and resilient structure.

Too often, environmental factors interact to prevent full expression of inherited bone-density potential.[1] Habits from infancy on may account for 23 percent of bone variability.[2] These factors include:
> Food choices
> Sports activities
> Combination of foods eaten at one meal
> Frequency of dieting
> Skipped meals

For females, bone mass accumulation by age twenty is also associated with maternal bone mass.

> **Hereditary contributions from your mother play an overwhelmingly critical role in your bone health.**

But nature is forgiving: Good environmental influences on bone consolidation during the decades before menopause may be more important in promoting optimal or peak bone mass, thereby helping to prevent or delay the postmenopausal onset of osteoporotic fractures.[3]

Until the time of menopause, bone mass is also enhanced by child-bearing and lactation; beyond menopause, environmental factors dominate.[4]

If you are an average healthy adult, you lose 500 milligrams of calcium from your bones every day.[5] That's half a gram! At that rate, your bones would be reduced to powder in just a few years. What saves your skeleton is the fact that 500 milligrams of calcium are deposited *back* into your bone structure daily. Special bone cells called *osteoblasts* take calcium and phosphorus from your blood and deposit crystals in your bone structure. But other cells, *osteoclasts*, remove those same crystals and return calcium and phosphorus to your blood plasma. The outer layer of your bones—the calcium phosphate—is the material subject to the actions of these cells. This is very convenient—it makes the calcium readily accessible when needed.

Why this seemingly risky interchange of bone material into and out of your bones? *Because it's extremely important for your body to preserve a specific concentration of calcium in your blood plasma.* The precise level of calcium is maintained even at the expense of the structural integrity of your bones because calcium is also responsible for:

- ➤ Nerve cell communication
- ➤ Contraction of muscle cells
- ➤ Blood-clotting efficiency
- ➤ Function of very important enzymes
- ➤ Production of certain life-supporting proteins

FIGURE 12

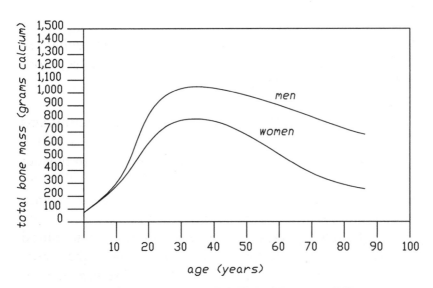

age (years)

RELATIONSHIP BETWEEN AGE AND BONE MASS IN THE U.S.

Men suffer from osteoporosis too, but the loss of bone mass is far more severe in women in this country. (In Hong Kong, as many men as women suffer from the disease. In Singapore, more men than women are afflicted.)

Total blood calcium must be carefully maintained at about 10 milligrams per 100 milliliters of plasma (about a quarter of a gram in an average adult woman). But calcium is continually being filtered out by your kidneys and excreted. As indicated, bone tissue is a natural place to store and retrieve calcium as required—to maintain the balance.

Can you get enough calcium for bone health from your dinner plate? *Not always, because dietary calcium is unreliable.* Note the following:

(1) **Intestinal absorption** of calcium supplied by food is never more than about 50 percent efficient.

(2) An excess of **fat** reduces calcium absorption.[6]

(3) Calcium absorption decreases with **age**, the decline starting earlier for women.[7]

(4) **Antacids, tetracyclines, laxatives, diuretics,** and other drugs impede calcium absorption.[8]

(5) **Individual differences** result in extreme variations. Example: calcium retention of two normal five-year-olds eating the same food was ex amined. One retained 78 percent more calcium than the other.[9]

(6) There is a direct correlation between **salt intake** and calcium excretion.

(7) **Chlorine** in tap water, soft drinks, and restaurant coffees and teas causes calcium excretion.

Bone is a specialized connective tissue. Together with cartilage, it makes up the skeleton. These tissues serve three functions. They are: (1) a mechanical support and site of muscle attachment for locomotion; (2) protection for vital organs and bone marrow; (3) a metabolic reserve of ions for the entire organism, especially for calcium and phosphorus

Phosphorus metabolism is driven by the same hormones that control calcium. This is understandable, since calcium and phosphorus are incorporated together into bone structure. But this assumes a ratio of calcium and phosphorus found in a natural diet. All too often, just as with sodium and potassium, we subject ourselves to an unbalanced ratio— caused by the excess phosphorus we consume with our sodas, meat products, cheese, baked goods, and other highly processed foods. *Too much phosphorus prevents the proper assimilation of new calcium into your bone tissue.* In addition, phosphorus levels are not as tightly controlled as calcium levels, so, unlike calcium, assimilation of phosphorus can skyrocket.

The concept that estrogen is a major factor in bone health is misleading. An article in *Bone* (1996,185S) points to the fact that the importance of menopause to the problems of osteoporosis has been overemphasized. The researchers state that the causes of osteoporosis are clearly not related to gonadal status, because these phenomena are observed both in men and in women. Targeting women at menopause for osteoporosis is not a helpful approach.

Confusion also centers around bone mass. One study shows that women with the greatest bone mass are more than twice as likely to develop breast cancer as women with the lowest bone mass because bone mass may reflect a woman's cumulative exposure to estrogen. These new findings may be "cause for concern if you have a family history of breast cancer, and are currently taking or considering taking estrogen replacement therapy," said Dr. Stanley Wallach, director of Endocrinology at the Osteoporosis Treatment Center at the Hospital for Joint Diseases in New York. "Taking estrogen can substantially increase bone mass in postmenopausal women." (The effect wears off, however, when treatment is stopped.)

FIGURE 13

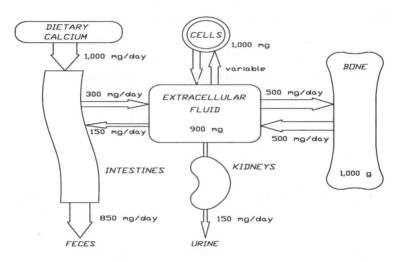

CALCIUM: IN AND OUT OF BONE

This represents the typical daily flow of calcium in and out of bone tissue. Less than a third of dietary calcium is absorbed.

~~~

The proportion of osteoporotic pelvic fractures increased from 18% in 1970 to 52% in 1991. The proportion of patients over 60 years of age increased from 28% in 1970 to a shocking 62% in 1991—increasing more rapidly than can be accounted for by the demographic changes only.

For a 50 year old caucasian women today, the risk of a hip fracture over her remaining lifetime is about 17%. Tomorrow the situation will clearly be worse because the continual increase in life expectancy will cause a 3-fold rise in worldwide fracture incidence over the next 60 years, particularly in women, but also in men. The cost of hip fracture is expected to dramaticaly increase in the next decades.

FIGURE 14

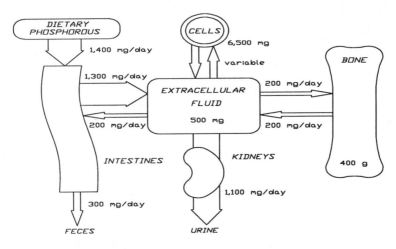

PHOSPHORUS: IN AND OUT OF BONE

This represents the typical daily flow of phosphorus in and out of bone tissue. Absorption is above 90 percent. Excessive dietary phosphorus can interfere with proper utilization of calcium.

~~~

The risk of institutionalization after hip fracture is high, partly explained by the *poor prefracture health status of many people who fracture their hips.*
> *Australian/New Zealand Public Health Journal* (1996 Dec;20:579)

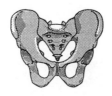

MEMOS

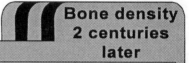

LEARNING ABOUT BONE DENSITY FROM COFFINS IN ENGLISH BURIAL CRYPTS

The incidence of osteoporotic hip fractures has been increasing faster than the rate expected if it were adjusted for life expectancy. The restoration of a London church, during which bone fragments dating from 1729 to 1852 were recovered, provided a novel opportunity to compare the occurrence of historical bone loss with that of present-day women.

Women suffer far greater bone loss today than two centuries ago, both pre- and postmenopausally. The researchers saw the typical decline in premenopausal bone density in present-day women but found no significant loss in these preserved samples. This suggests that a 70-year-old woman today would have a lower bone density than a 70-year-old woman who had lived two centuries ago.

Lancet, 1993[10]

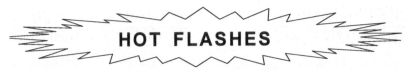

HOT FLASHES

➤ A maternal history of hip fracture doubles risk. Weight gain after age 25 lowers risk. Spending fewer than 4 hours a day on your feet increases risk. Walking for exercise reduces risk.

New England Jnl of Medicine, 1995[11]

➤ Low hipbone density is a stronger predictor of hip fracture than bone density at other sites.

Lancet, 1993[12]

➤ The more caffeine, the more bone loss.

Epidemiology, 1993[13]

➤ The development of optimal bone mass early in life is more effective in preventing osteoporosis than traditional measures used later in life.

Clinical Rheumatology, 1989[14]

Osteoporosis International, 1990[15]

➤ After menopause, environmental factors override the advantages of reproductive and breast-feeding history for bone mineral density.

American Jnl of Epidemiology, 1992[16]

➤ After age 30 to 35, the total amount of bone shrinks about 10 percent per decade in women.
and about 5 percent per decade in men. Women over 55 and men over 60 usually have had enough bone loss to produce at least one break.

Geriatrics, 1974[17]

➤ One of every six white women will have a hip fracture during her lifetime.

New England Jnl of Medicine, 1995[18]

➤ White women of small stature are at greatest risk for osteoporosis.

Startling New Facts About Osteoporosis, 1992[19]

➤ The reduction of bone mass with age is significantly greater in alcoholics, especially after age sixty.

Clinical Orthopedics & Related Research, 1973[20]

➤ *Any* dysfunction of *any* regulatory system can lead to changes in bone formation or resorption, and ultimately to skeletal disease.

British Dental Jnl, 1992[21]

➤ Cadmium concentrations in Pecos Indian bones were 50 times lower than today's humans.

Environmental Health Perspectives, 1991[22]

➤ The percentage of total body lead found in bones can range from 78 percent at age 20 to 96 percent at age 80, placing a burden on the body's bone health as we age.

Environmental Research, 1990[23]

➤ The osteoblasts can't make new bone unless the osteoclasts have done their work to provide the necessary space.

Optimal Health Guidelines, 1990[24]

➤ Although breast-feeding temporarily decreases bone mass, it doesn't increase risk of hip fracture.

New England Jnl of Medicine, 1995[25]

UPDATES

Acta Obstet Gynecol Scand 1997 Mar;76(3):189-99
The effect of HRT on bone mass wears off after discontinuation of treatment.

Arterioscler Thromb Vasc Biol 1997 Apr;17(4):680-7
Atherosclerotic calcification and osteoporosis often coexist. Research suggests that specific oxidized lipids may be the common factors underlying the pathogenesis of both atherosclerotic calcification and osteoporosis.

J Am Diet Assoc 1997 Apr;97(4):414-7
Osteoporosis is a disease of bone fragility that afflicts more than 25 million Americans and costs the economy of the United States approximately $13.8 billion per year. In addition to direct economic costs, osteoporosis frequently costs patients their independence and a decrease in quality of life.

~~ ENDNOTES ~~ *The fantasy continues...*

Back in our fantasy, we see exchanges taking place between bones and blood. The number of trades dwarf the total transactions made on the floor of the stock market on its busiest day. Instead of brokers directing the responses, hormones are calling the shots.

We see hormones moving calcium into our blood from two places—intestines and bones. We jump back quickly to get out of the way of the darting messages sent to these two warehouses—signals to release their calcium inventory into our blood. We observe the more important aspects—those that influence calcium's deposition, storage, transportation, and arrival at key locations. We are impressed by the complicated internal traffic control systems manipulated by the hormones.

Now it's obvious that estrogen is not the sole regulator of these transactions. This private network is dependent on more than just one hormone.

Even more fascinating, we see that the constant inflow and outflow of bone materials also allows for bone modification in response to individual changing requirements. It allows our bones to thicken and strengthen when we exercise regularly, and to heal after they break. Now we know that bone is living tissue, and that it can be compressed with surprising, maybe even *alarming*, facility.

"Look at all those green vegetables. I want you to eat them so your bones will look good in a big museum some day!"

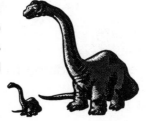

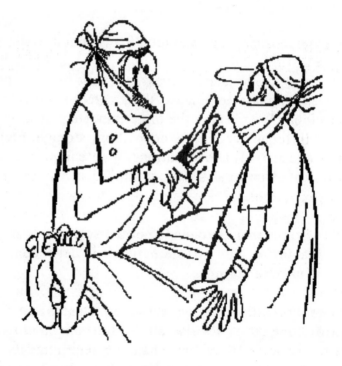

It's going to rain.
I can feel it in her bones.

Reprinted from *Startling New Facts About Osteoporosis*
by Betty Kamen, Nutrition Encounter, Inc., 1992

7

BONE AND SEX HORMONES

SO WHAT DO SEX HORMONES HAVE TO DO WITH BONES?

What do sex hormones have to do with bones? Good question! The problem is that we don't really know more than a small part of the answer. "Key ingredients of osteoporosis pathophysiology are missing from the prevailing understanding,"[1] to use language of the technical journals.

> We do know that natural progesterone stimulates the growth and spread of osteoblasts,[2] and that other sex steroids play a role in the physiology of bone![3]

In more general terms, we know that serious loss of bone mass is closely correlated with menopause. During the first six years following its onset, the decrease in mineral density of some of our bones can be *three to ten times higher than the change in the decade prior to menopause.*[4] And the biggest change in menopause is the decline of steroid hormones!

Therefore, it has been logical to assume that artificially replacing the lost hormones could have a beneficial effect on bone strength. In fact it does—sort of. Synthetic estrogen, used as estrogen replacement therapy (abbreviated ERT, or more recently, HRT for hormone replacement therapy), has been reported to reduce the rate of bone loss[5] and to decrease the incidence of bone fractures by 50 percent.[6] If this is so, why is controversy so prevalent?

For starters, not every researcher gets the same result. In one extensive study spanning 14 years, no decrease in hip fractures could be detected with the use of ERT.[7] Another study shows no advantage in bone protection from ERT once a woman reaches age 75. But let's allow the benefit of doubt and assume that fractures really can be reduced by 50 percent. This would be a compelling statistic, but the fracture rate would still be too high and too devastating for too many women.

If the dilemma of osteoporosis were addressed effectively, there would be almost *no* fractures! Aside from a rare accident, older women simply do not subject their bones to stresses that should cause them to break. Twisting your foot the wrong way as you step down a curb or straining to open a window should not cause a fracture! And how many skydiving senior citizens do you know?

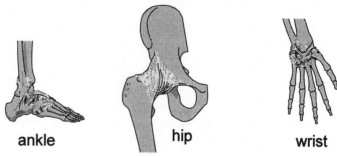

ankle   hip   wrist

Common breaking points

> Currently, there are 1,500,000 fractures every year attributable to osteoporosis.[8]

Even if we could treat all women who might benefit—reducing the number of fractures to 750,000—we'd still have a big problem. And that's now. The number of women aged 65 and older is expected to double by the year 2000![9]

According to a report by the Study of Osteoporotic Fractures Research Group (a combined effort of major university hospitals including more than 8,000 women), *the decline in steroid hormones with age does not entirely account for the increasing risk of hip fractures.* Environmental exposures play a large role, as do cigarette smoking, caffeine intake, use of long-acting sedatives, inactivity, and reduced body weight. We are putting our eggs in one basket when we focus on sex-hormone deficiencies alone as the causative factor for broken bones.[10]

Here's another intriguing fact: tamoxifen is an anti-estrogen drug given to breast-cancer prone women to block the uptake of estrogen hormones. If lack of estrogen is the cause of osteoporosis, one would expect tamoxifen to cause bone density loss. But tamoxifen does no such thing![11]

So decreased hormonal output is not the only cause of bone density loss. Nor is bone density loss the only cause of broken bones. Lower hormonal production is, however, a significant contributing factor.

There is no question that *osteoporosis is a preventable and treatable condition.*

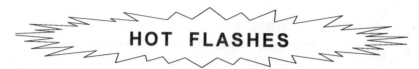

HOT FLASHES

➤ Osteoporotic fractures have an enormous impact on mortality, productivity, independence, and self-esteem. They are the most important causes of ill health and death among older people.

New England Jnl of Medicine, 1995[12]

➤ Adult women face a 17.5 percent lifetime risk of of a hip fracture, costing $45 billion in the next ten years.

Bone, 1994[13]

➤ People with chronic bronchitis who are treated with corticosteroids—even at low doses—are at risk for osteoporosis.

Osteoporosis International, 1992[14]

➤ Bone loss can be caused by *acidosis*. Acidosis occurs for many reasons, including poor breathing (as in bronchitis).

John Lee, M.D., 1993[15]

➤ Even in the first postmenopausal decade, osteoporotic women have low spine bone mineral density, small vertebral area, and low body weight. Such women are at risk of crush fracture.

Jnl of Bone and Mineral Research, 1994[16]

➤ The rate of broken bones increased in females twice as fast as population growth.

Geriatrics, 1974[17]

UPDATES

Int J Epidemiol 1996 Apr;25(2):403-10
Dietary factors have an influence on bone mass, thereby affecting fracture susceptibility.

J Am Coll Nutr 1996 Dec;15(6):556-69
Skeletal modeling results from a complex sequence of hormonal changes in interaction with nutritional factors.

~~ ENDNOTES ~~ *The fantasy continues...*

As we re-enter our fantasy, some of us are amazed at the ongoing battles. Others are familiar with the clashes and know about enemy cells trying to get the upper hand. Immune cells intercede—a never-ending process in our seemingly healthy body. Most of us know that cells carrying seeds of damage can be overpowered and attacked by immune warriors endowed with killer status, but we had no idea how frequently it happens. It is so much a part of everyday life!

The ending is not always a happy one. The corrupt cell can split, unchallenged, and become two, then four, then eight. When proliferation is out of control, we call it *cancer*.

In our fantasy, the difference between cell death and cell murder is very clearly defined. What did *you* have for dinner last night? ("We have met the enemy and it is us.") We watch as *synthetic* hormones attempt to play real-life roles. (There goes the neighborhood.) Try as they will, they cannot imitate. No Oscar Award here—*the performance of the look-alike stuff just isn't good enough.*

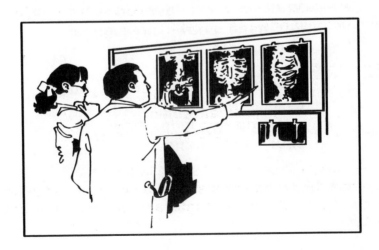

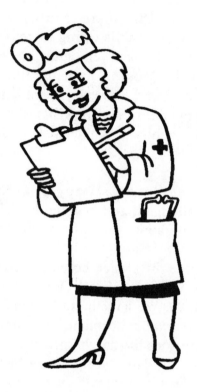

Your index finger on your left hand shows no sign of osteoporosis.

Now I'm going to refer you to a colleague who will examine the index finger on your right hand.

8

SEX HORMONES AND CANCER AND OTHER SIDE EFFECTS

WHAT ABOUT SEX HORMONES AND CANCER?

Then there's the cancer risk. Perhaps more than any other disease, we have come to regard cancer as the Grim Reaper of our time. But the process that makes a cell cancerous is the same process by which a cell grows, replicates, and propagates. Cancer could be thought of as a group of cells overperforming.

The built-in control mechanism that tells a cell to stop multiplying has somehow gotten its signals crossed. The result is runaway cell growth that can eventually have severe consequences. And yet, overproduction seems to be found everywhere in development, followed by "a pruning back of the branches of surviving cells," as William Calvin, neurobiologist and professor at the University of Washington, author of *In Search Of The Brain's Voice*, explains: *"All you need for cancer is failure to prune.* What's interesting about this is the unusual growth and control that's going on all over your body all the time. Perhaps there's really no such thing as perfect health, just periods of time when all this microscopic backing and filling is hidden from view."[1]

As long as intercellular signalling and immune systems function well, cancer remains under control in a healthy body. Many substances promote or accelerate cell growth and many more help to control it. Estrogen encourages growth. It is referred to as "the hormone for beginnings," or, "the hormone of life." This conveys an idea of the power of estrogen but also its danger in the context of cancer.

There is no question that excessive estrogen may increase the risk of endometrial cancer (cancer of the lining of the uterus).[2] The National Institutes of Health Consensus Development Conference on Osteoporosis issued an official statement concerning endometrial cancer and ERT, informing women that estrogen therapy places women at high risk. Although the conference acknowledged the high risk of estrogen therapy, it suggested that there was no need for concern, making an outrageous (in my opinion) statement about its possible side effect: "Estrogen-associated endometrial cancer is usually manifested at an early stage and is rarely fatal when managed appropriately."[3] Great. It's okay if you get cancer—then the good doctor can zap you with radiation and chemotherapy to keep you from dying.

Research varies as to whether or not estradiol and estrone (forms of estrogen) cause tumors and cancer.[4] Controversy often stems from lack of consideration of excesses and/or synthetic forms of these hormones. *We must understand that estrogens don't initiate cancer; they can, however, promote it.*

Remember DES, a synthetic estrogen used between 1945 and 1971 to help prevent miscarriages—**despite the fact that we knew since the 1930s that it was carcinogenic?** There's a tragically high risk of vaginal cancer in girls whose mothers had DES treatment during pregnancy.

Males in utero exposed to DES developed with undescended testicles. They may be less masculine, too, because the undescended testicle interrupts the production of testosterone. Newest findings report that these males also have decreased semen volume and sperm counts. There is even evidence that exposed females may be masculinized.[5] Turns out it was a useless and needless drug anyway, never promoting the promised results.

A little known fact is that women were also given DES after the birth of their babies to dry their milk production because they were discouraged from breastfeeding. It didn't work in this capacity, either. A report in *Molecular Carcinogens* (1996;15:115) explains how DES causes an *alteration in gene expression*, which often occurs in estrogen-related malignancies.

Does it anger you to know that DES was allowed to be used *forty years* after its cancer-causing potential had been discovered? I anticipate the same history for the estrogen/progestin scenario! You can see that when hormone balances are askew, powerful influences come into play.[6] Do you really want to artificially promote the "capacity for growth" in your tissues?

Although there is little doubt that estrogens are potent mammary tumor promoters when present in surplus amounts, these actions are poorly understood.[7] Studies also support the notion that female hormones—when superfluous and synthetic—play a role in the development of brain tumors.[8] Allowing drugs to be used in light of horrendous side effects is, sadly, nothing new.

Because women can become pregnant during the few years prior to menopause, starting any kind of synthetic hormone therapy too early must be considered with extreme caution.

FOOD SOURCES OF HORMONES

A mounting body of evidence suggests that sources of hormones in our food environment contribute to the background level of carcinogens. Hormones are implanted in the ears of 90 percent of feedlot animals. Consequently, milk, commercial eggs, and other dairy products have traces of these hormones. Most commercial-grade meat is laced with it; birth control pills are based on it—all piled on top of other carcinogens accumulating in our environment.

Veterinary drugs have been regarded as necessary to produce food of animal origin. The drug residues create problems associated with the use of these hormonal or hormone-related compounds endowed with growth-promoting properties. It's difficult to monitor excessive use. Tests are not sophisticated enough to discern differences between the animals' own production of natural hormones and those added by the industry.

According to a published review of drug practices in animals, the current use of hormone compounds for "improved" food production does not rest on solid scientific ground.[9]

So keep in mind that when you buy a bottle of milk, it usually comes from a cow that has been given growth hormone to enhance its milk yield.[10] Hormones from the hypothalamus, pituitary, thyroid, adrenals, pancreas, and gonads, as well as related substances such as prostaglandins and growth factors, have been detected in milk. Prolactin in milk consumed by a pregnant woman may have deleterious long-term effects on mammary glands of her offspring. It may also retard the preweaning growth, hasten puberty, control certain neuronal activity, and influence the fluid absorption of the children.[11]

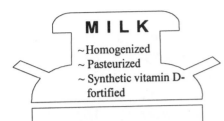

MILK

~ Homogenized
~ Pasteurized
~ Synthetic vitamin D-
fortified

This product may be hazardous to your health!

Many foods promoted as healthful are highly processed and may not be in your best health interest.

URGENT REPORTS

1996 Medical Tribune News Service

"Exposure to toxic chemicals in the environment is thought to be disruptive to the hormones of animals, resulting in reproductive and other changes. A chemical spill in a lake near Orlando, Fla., may be the reason that resident male alligators have hormone levels similar to females. Various cancers, including those of the breast, prostate and testicles, also have risen in the past few decades."

Clinical Chemistry 1995 Dec;41(12 Pt 2): 1896-901

"Male reproductive health has been declining. Treatment of several million pregnant women with the synthetic estrogen, diethylstilbestrol, led to an increase in these conditions among the sons of these women. We speculate that alteration in exposure to estrogen in the past half-century may have caused the changes in male reproductive health."

Drug Safety 1996 Nov;15(5):360-70

"There is an increased incidence of breast cancer after long-term hormone replacement therapy."

Manipulation of fatty acid profiles in cows is a common practice in our effort to produce lean meat. Biologically active residues frequently result from illegal treatment of animals sold for food in the marketplace![12] You are protected to a small extent by the FDA and your liver. What? The FDA and your liver? Yes, but neither has what it takes for total command—that is, the FDA doesn't have sufficient police power to examine *all* markets, and chances are *you* don't have all the nutrients necessary for *first-pass removal* by your liver.

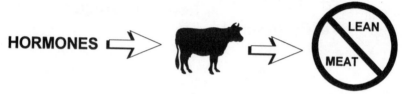

Commentary on the possible effect of hormones in food on human growth was reported in *Medical Hypotheses*. According to studies noted by Dr. N. Moishezon-Blank, the practice of adding hormones to food may render your liver incapable of efficient first-pass removal.

Changes in the shape and size of young Americans' heads show a tendency toward a decrease in size! Moishezon-Blank and colleagues suggest that the general acceleration of growth in the most recent American generation could be caused by accumulated hormone residues in the diet. Affecting long bones more than any other tissue, these residues also trigger inhibitors of growth during earlier stages of flat bone development. Consequently, the relative size of the skull (a flat bone structure), with respect to the body, is diminished. A reduction in the absolute size of the skull as well may accompany the change of body/head proportion.[13] Wouldn't you like to see more studies to validate these observations?

> Hormone residues in milk may contribute to the increased height of the new generation of Asian Americans.

It should be noted that *estriol—the kind of estrogen that the placenta produces*—does not appear to be carcinogenic. This hormone may even have protective effects.[14] A healthy liver converts estrone and estradiol to estriol, but the conversion may not always be complete. A significant amount of the potentially harmful forms of estrogen may get through. The safe form (that is, the estriol) is available for therapeutic purposes.

Although today's medical journals advocate hormone replacement therapy for all women, occasionally a more balanced view appears. The *International Journal Of Fertility* proclaimed the following:

> *Not all postmenopausal women need estrogen replacement. Some continue to produce significant amounts of their own estrogens.[15]*

When you read or are told about safety features of "new" hormone therapies, remember that the results are usually being compared with their more harmful counterparts currently or formerly in use, rather than with natural modalities.

> Remember, too, that short-term experiments are never as meaningful as studies spanning the years—especially when hormones are involved.

MORE ABOUT ERT AND SIDE EFFECTS

Possible (if not usual) side effects of ERT:
        Abdominal cramps
        Amenorrhea
        Bloating
        Breast tenderness and enlargement
        Cystitis-like syndromes
        Elevated blood pressure
        Endometrial cancer
        Gallbladder disease
        Hair loss (where you don't want it)
        Hair growth (where you don't want it)
        Hyperlipidemia
        Jaundice
        Loss of libido
        Mental depression
        Nausea and vomiting
        Prolonged vaginal bleeding
        Reduced carbohydrate tolerance
        Reduced glucose tolerance
        Skin rashes
        Thrombophlebitis
        Undesirable weight gain
        Vaginal candidiasis[16,17,18]

Reflect on this list. Then note this quotation from the pages of *Senior Patient*, a subsidiary of *Postgraduate Medicine*:

> *It now seems reasonable to recommend that <u>all</u> postmenopausal women—regardless of age or symptoms—be seriously considered for hormone replacement therapy. The disadvantages are not necessarily medically risky, but are a matter of patients' attitudes.*[19]

Huh? A matter of *attitude*? Here we go again!

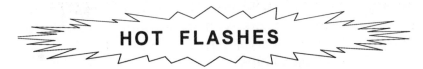

HOT FLASHES

➢ Risks of estrogen therapy include endometrial cancer, breast cancer, and gallstones.

American Heart Jnl, 1994[20]

➢ A Western diet elevates levels of sex hormones, increasing harmful steroids and decreasing formation of mammalian compounds which could protect against cancer cell growth.

Scandinavian Jnl of Clin & Lab Invest, 1990[21]

➢ ERT increases risk of endometrial cancer during treatment and years after it is discontinued.

Obstetrics and Gynecology, 1990[22]

➢ Evidence supporting estrogen's role in breast cancer comes from international studies.

Breast Cancer Research and Treatment, 1991[23]

➢ Synthetic progestins induce proliferation of breast tumor cells.

Molecular and Cellular Endocrinology, 1994[24]

➢ Cervical cancer is stimulated in response to excess estradiol.

International Jnl of Cancer, 1992[25]

➢ Estrogen contributes to gallbladder cancer.

Medical Hypotheses, 1991[26]

➢ Estradiol-17 beta is associated with breast cancer.

Breast Cancer Research and Treatment, 1992[27]

➢ Lab studies suggest that some androgenic hormones stimulate cancer in bladder tissue.

Cancer Causes and Control, 1992[28]

➢ Sex hormones may have a role in broncho- genic carcinoma.

Cancer Research, 1990[29]

➢ The potential for pancreatic cancer can be demonstrated after hormonal manipulations.

International Jnl of Pancreatology, 1990[30]

> Significant stimulation of certain gastric and colorectal cells occurs with large concentrations of estradiol.

Cancer, 1989[31]

> Estrogen therapy may contribute to breast cancer because the mammary gland is already oversaturated with estrogens.

Revue Francaise de Gyn et D Obstetrique, 1991[32]

> There is direct evidence of a relationship between lowered spatial ability and prenatal exposure to DES in males.

Hormones and Behavior, 1992[33]

> To evaluate its effects on the endometrium, biopsy is essential with progestin therapy. This biopsy is associated with pain and discomfort.

Maturitas, 1994[34]

UPDATES

Cancer Epidemiol Biomarkers Prev 1997 Jan;6(1):11-4
The relationship between HRT and breast cancer risk is particularly critical for women continuing to use HRT several years after menopause.

JAMA 1996 Feb 7;275(5):370-5
Daily doses of estrogen enhance the development of endometrial hyperplasia.

Tidsskr Nor Laegeforen 1997 Apr 20;117(10):1493-5
Recent studies demonstrate a higher risk of endometrium cancer in breast cancer patients treated with tamoxifen, and higher risk of abnomalities in the endometrium in healthy women. **Prevention trials, when tamoxifen is given to healthy women, are disputed, owing to the apparent carcinogenic effect of tamoxifen.**

1996 Medical Tribune News Service
Tamoxifen has been associated with an increased risk of cancers in breast cancer patients. Longer use is associated with increased risk of endometrial cancer.

~~ ENDNOTES ~~ *The fantasy continues...*

We affirm that hormone therapy could, for a time, slow the process of bone loss, but there are risks involved.

Our fantasy reveals an exciting surprise! We didn't think we could rebuild bone once osteoporosis left its calling card. But look at those osteoblasts—they're gobbling up all that progesterone and *empowering new bone construction—enough to make up for longtime deprivation!* It's a slow process, like watching grass grow—but it is happening.

If we put our fantasy on fast forward, we can actually see it occur—*but not to those without the progesterone.* See how much more efficiently bone growth comes about when we add special nutrients.

And look! It's even happening to that much older woman. Wow!

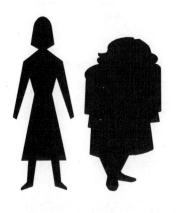

One of the first symptoms of osteoporosis may be loss of height. The progressive decrease in bone mass results in this gradual decline *and eventual "dowager's hump," known as* kyphosis. *The hunchback look is caused by the abnormally* increased convex shape in the spine's curvature.

IT DOESN'T HAVE TO BE THIS WAY!

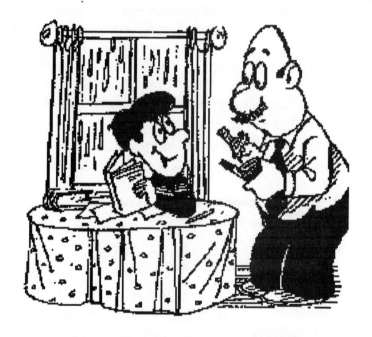

Hurry up and bring me a glass
of wine before my doctor changes
his mind about it.

9

NATURAL PROGESTERONE

A BETTER HORMONE FOR REPLACEMENT

The dangers of estrogen replacement therapy are only part of the problem. *Early researchers were not looking at all the facts.* No one paid much attention to the research showing that progesterone tapers off at about the same time that the process of osteoporosis begins, followed years later by the decline of estrogen.

> "There seems to be no good reason to have chosen estrogen over progesterone as the hormone of replacement. The decline of progesterone, beginning several years before menopause when estrogen sufficiency persists, correlates better than estrogen with the onset of osteoporosis."

The statement above was made by John R. Lee, MD, a retired physician in northern California who has had significant success reversing osteoporosis in his patients. He has been a pioneer in the use of natural progesterone.[1]

But we still strive for facts which are more than "guilt by association." We need to understand just what estrogen and progesterone are doing to our bones, and awareness has finally surfaced. Jerilynn Prior, MD, of the Endocrinology and Metabolism Division of the University of British Columbia, identified the roles of these hormones in bone remodelling. Estrogen reduces the rate of bone loss by reducing the activity of *osteoclasts*, the cells that *resorb* calcium phosphate back into our blood plasma. (Resorption refers to calcium leaving our bone and reentering our blood.) Progesterone, on the other hand, actually works in conjunction with *osteoblasts*, the cells associated with building new bone material, as described earlier.

Typical of so many revelations, Dr. Prior's awareness of progesterone's role in bone health came about accidentally. She was measuring the estrogen and progesterone levels of female athletes. The results were unrelated to her expectations; she discovered that the athletes who had low progesterone but high estrogen levels showed signs of osteoporosis. How could this be? Wasn't it an established fact that *estrogen* deficiency causes osteoporosis? Could this mean that *progesterone* deficiency is the culprit?

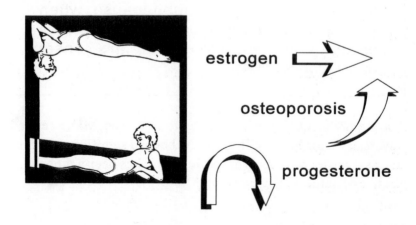

Prior's suspicions were confirmed. She explains:

Progesterone binds to receptors on osteo-blasts, increases the rate of bone formation and remodelling when given therapeutically to oophorectomized dogs [dogs whose ova-ries are removed], and slows bone loss in postmenopausal women. Progesterone acts on bone, even though estrogen activity is low or absent. Because progesterone appears to work on the osteoblast to increase bone formation, it would complement the actions of estrogen to decrease bone resorption.[2]

In other words, progesterone builds bone!

Dr. Prior cites additional validation in a letter published in the *New England Journal of Medicine*:

Evidence that progesterone acts as a bone-trophic [stimulating] hormone has been ex-tended by work documenting the presence of progesterone receptors on osteoblasts.[3]

Studies on both animals and humans show that progesterone has a growth-promoting effect on bone tissue. Research with nonmenopausal women treated with *natural proges-terone* suggests that such a hormone might prevent bone loss![4] This explains why ERT alone yields limited results. Estrogen can reduce the rate of bone loss, but bone loss is only one problem. In view of the risks, doesn't it make more sense to work on supplying more *new bone material* instead of just reducing the rate of bone loss? (It's one thing to spend less money and slow the decline of your bank account. It's quite another to replace the money to keep the balance stable.)

Dr. Lee validates these results clinically. He recounts success in actually *reversing* osteoporosis, instead of merely arresting its progress. This excerpt is from his paper published in *Medical Hypothesis*, summarizing the outcome of his treatment plan:

> *Since 1982, I have followed 100 patients, all postmenopausal white women (average age 65.2 years, range 38 to 83 years) in a suburban setting. The average time from menopause was 16 years. The majority had already noted height loss, a cardinal sign of osteoporosis, and many had experienced one or more fractures. The benefits from the treatment program were so obvious to these patients that no problems with patient compliance arose. Nor were any side effects or adverse alterations in blood lipids observed. Each patient was followed a minimum of three years.*
>
> *In the study group of 100 patients, height loss was stabilized, previous musculoskeletal aches and pains disappeared, and no osteoporotic fractures occurred. Three traumatic fractures did occur and, in each case, these healed normally with the treating orthopedist commenting on the good quality of [the patients'] bones.*
>
> *In the major sub-group of 63 patients with...bone density tests, the average three-year change in density actually increased 15.4 percent, instead of losing an expected 4.5 percent.[5]*

One must be impressed with Dr. Lee's human trials and their encouraging outcomes. They strongly suggest that osteoporosis can be reversed. Dr. Lee found that age did not seem to be a determinant—even 70-year-old patients experienced the same increase in bone density as younger women. As is usually the case with adaptogenic natural treatments—rather than symptom-suppressing synthetic therapies—those with the lowest bone densities experienced the *greatest* relative improvement. (See Table 2 below.)

TABLE 2
DR. LEE'S DATA:
BONE DENSITY IMPROVEMENT
WITH PROGESTERONE

Lumbar Bone Mass Density (gm/sq cm)	Initial Average	3-Year Average	% Gain
0.5-0.8	0.745	0.911	22.8
0.8-0.9	0.838	0.992	18.4
0.9-1.0	0.957	1.122	17.2
1.0-1.1	1.026	1.134	10.5
1.1-1.2	1.152	1.215	5.5
1.2-1.3	1.256	1.289	2.6

What did Dr. Lee do to achieve his remarkable success? Diet, supplements, exercise, and natural progesterone were part of the blueprint. Dietary changes emphasized leafy greens as a calcium source rather than traditional dairy products. This makes sense in view of the high incidence of lactose intolerance (inability to digest milk sugars), a problem that intensifies as we get older. (Blacks and Asians face this problem in their teens; northern Europeans as adults.)

Red meat was limited, sodas avoided, cigarettes not allowed at all, and alcohol severely curbed.

The daily supplements included:
- ➤ 350-400 IU vitamin D
- ➤ 2,000 milligrams vitamin C
- ➤ 25,000 IU beta-carotene (a vitamin A precursor)
- ➤ 800-1,000 milligrams calcium (See Chapter 10 for updated specifics on calcium supplements and why doses do not have to be as high.)

0.3 to 0.625 milligrams per day of conjugated estrogen was taken for three weeks each month. [Conjugated estrogen is a mixture of estrogenic substances of the type excreted by pregnant mares, as in Premarin—"conjugated" to enhance absorption. (Today, there are safer forms of estrogen recommended by nutrition-oriented MDs, prescribed only when necessary—and then only for a short period of time.)

Natural progesterone in a cream base was applied to the skin under the arms, on the neck, breasts, belly, and face (alternately) before bed, twelve days during the last two weeks of monthly estrogen use.

Except for the estrogen and progesterone, this regimen is perfectly sensible for virtually anybody who wants to improve overall health. Dr. Lee's dietary suggestions are similar to those I've been trying to get my family and friends to abide by for most of my life!

Since Dr. Lee's initial work, new creams in the marketplace have sprung up. Successful varieties contain the extract of Mexican wild yam, low doses of progesterone, and several synergistic herbs, including Siberian ginseng, black cohosh, and burdock root. These herbs allow for even more effectiveness with lower doses of progesterone. Creams may also include a few or all of the following oils: almond, safflower, avocado, and jojoba. The oils are present for several reasons, including better delivery into your bloodstream. Aloe vera and chamomile may also be added.

Long-term estrogen therapy is not easy, as confirmed by the high degree of noncompliance among women who start the drug, and give up because of unpleasant side effects.[6] Again: unlike estrogen therapy, the application of natural progesterone in a cream base has met with incredible success.

Dr. Lee acknowledges the absence of a control group or double-blind studies at the early stages of natural progesterone use. He points out, however, that conventional treatment programs—those using estrogen alone—are a kind of *real-world* control group. Results with synthetic hormones have been anything but positive, especially in terms of risk. The good news is that we now have an enormous global basis for judgment: *Overwhelming success stories have been reported with the use of natural progesterone creams, especially those containing synergistic herbs.*

Studies indicating that synthetic progestin may have a bone-restoring effect have presented complications. For example, double-blind, placebo-controlled research involving postmenopausal women over a two-year time period showed that while overall bone loss was no greater for a progestin-only group, certain specific bone tissues seemed to lose less material with the use of estrogen only.[7,8]

Another similar study by the same researchers demonstrated synthetic progestin alone to be equivalent to estrogen alone. In Dr. Prior's clinical observations of postmenopausal women with endocrine disorders (that precluded estrogen treatment), patients all experienced an increase in vertebral bone density after one year on medroxyprogesterone.[9] (Medroxyprogesterone is the widely used synthetic progesterone, as in Provera.)

It is more than likely that the test results of these studies would have been even more dramatic if not for one factor: *the research included the use of oral, synthetic progestins.* Recall that outside sources of hormones are subject to destruction on the first pass through your liver. The natural *transdermal* form is the best way to bypass this roadblock. In his book, *Nutrition for Women*, biologist Raymond Peat, PhD, of Eugene, Oregon, advocates the transdermal method of administering progesterone as superior to oral, injection, suppository, or sublingual methods.[10]

An interesting study by Joel Hargrove, MD, of the Obstetrics and Gynecology Department of Vanderbuilt University Medical Center, compares the use of natural progesterone and estradiol with that of synthetic progestin (medroxyprogesterone acetate) and conjugated estrogens.[11] Women sought treatment for symptoms related to menopause and volunteered for a 12-month study. Results are shown in Table 3 on page 117.

Despite the information cited consistently across medical publications about the so-called "advantages" of adding progestins to estrogen therapy, many physicians in this country still prescribe unopposed estrogen![12] (Unopposed estrogen refers to the use of estrogen without the balance of progesterone— synthetic *or* natural.) Furthermore, the physicians who even *think* of checking for progesterone levels are few and far between.

Martin Milner, a naturopathic physician in Portland, Oregon, reports that not a single patient complaining of PMS or menopausal symptoms ever had a progesterone level determined by any of the physicians they had consulted before coming to his office.[13] (Dr. Milner has been in practice about 18 years.)

TABLE 3
COMPARISON OF TWO THERAPIES
Estradiol with Progesterone
and
Conjugated Estrogens with Medroxyprogesterone

Symptoms	Estradiol and Natural Progesterone		Conjugated Estrogens and Medroxyprogesterone	
	Baseline (before treatment)	12 months later	Baseline (before treatment)	12 months later
Hot flashes	9	0	5	3
Night sweats	6	0	4	3
Insomnia	4	1	3	1
Decreased libido	6	0	2	0
Vaginal dryness	5	0	3	2
Anxiety	6	3	3	1
Depression	1	1	3	0

Another impressive success rate! Look at the difference between the results of the two treatments. The combination of natural progesterone and estradiol is noticeably more effective than the more traditional mix of conjugated estrogen and medroxyprogesterone acetate.

So it's not always enough to talk about estrogen and progesterone. One must be very specific about the *form* in which these substances are administered. Of course, the study makes no attempt to determine which of the two variables in each part of the test was the more important—the natural progesterone or the estradiol; the synthetic progestin or the conjugated estrogen. I have my suspicions, but we await additional hard data from clinical trials.

The very latest research indicates that adding progestins to hormone replacement therapy increases the risk of breast cancer. And again the science goes unheeded—the newest trend is to prescribe a single pill for women, one containing *both* synthetic estrogen and synthetic progestins. The misdirected attitude is:

> *Let's make it easy for women to get both risk-laden drugs in one fell swoop!*

Other research validates the positive effects of natural progesterone supplementation. Examples follow.

➤ *Jnl of Steroid Biochem & Mol Biology*, 1996(58:72)
Progesterone promotes myelin formation in nerves of test animals. [Just think about the benefits this may have for multiple sclerosis patients!]

➤ *Endocrinology*, 1996(137:749-54)
Progesterone inhibits superoxide radical production.

➤ *Experimental Neurology*, 1996(138:246-51)
Progesterone decreases brain edema.

➤ *Jnl of Steroid Biochem & Mol Biology*, 1996(56:209)
Progesterone and its metabolites help to regulate estrogen receptors and to modulate uterine contractility.

➤ *Journal of Gynecology & Obstetrics*, 1980(18:444)
Uterine bleeding in the second trimester of pregnancy may be associated with low circulating levels of progesterone.

➤ *Journal of Obstetrics & Gynecology*, 1995(21:31-6)
Progesterone might intensify bone formation and suppress bone resorption.

➢ *Journal of Veterinary Medical Science*, 1995(57:845)
Measurement of progesterone is used as a potential noninvasive method to assess reproductive status in animals.

➢ Medical Tribune News Service, March 15, 1996
Men with higher levels of DHEA are less likely to have heart disease than those with lower levels. [Note: Use of progesterone cream may help to increase DHEA levels naturally.]

➢ *Eur Jnl Obstet Bynecol Reprod Biol* 1996(666:99)
Progesterone treatments are used for fibromas.

➢ *Clinical Obstetrics & Gynecology 1996(39:424)*
There is mounting evidence that progesterone is an essential component of the ovulatory process. Progesterone in preovulatory follicles are necessary for ovulation. Our knowledge of progesterone function has increased dramatically during the past decade.

➢ *Schweiz Rundsch Med Prax* 1995(84:127)
Applying progesterone vaginally leads to significantly higher concentrations and has effects on the uterine mucosa similar to those in a normal cycle.

➢ *Human Reproduction* 1996(11:980)
Progesterone may be important in the treatment regimens for women with immunological and endocrinological reproductive failure.

➢ *International Journal of Fertility*, 1987(18:444-7)
Supplementation of progesterone beginning in the luteal phase could reduce the risk of spontaneous abortions.

Natural progesterone:
~ acts as a regulator for the entire endocrine system
~ is also manufactured by the testes in males and adrenal cortex in males and females
~ helps to regulate accessory organs during the menstrual cycle
~ prepares the uterus for the implantation of the embryo by contributing to suppleness and circulation
~ helps to maintain pregnancy
~ has LDL cholesterol as its precursor in the luteal tissue
~ is secreted by the corpus luteum following the discharge of the ovum if no fertilization takes place
~ has a greater positive effect on bone-building in postmenopausal women than progestins
~ falls abruptly 10 to 12 days after ovulation, followed by the onset of menstruation
~ rises to 300 milligrams a day (by the placenta) during the third trimester
~ is carried in the blood by binding with cortisol-binding globulin
~ can be measured to confirm ovulation
~ can be a determinant for luteal function
~ has specific functions not found in any other compound
~ may reach a production rate during the luteal phase of 30 milligrams a day

~ can be produced synthetically and is
then called progestin, gestagen, or a
progestational agent
~ shares only the ability to sustain human
secretory endometrium with synthetic
progestogens (no synthetic progesterone has the full spectrum of natural
progesterone's biologic activity)
~ is not the same as synthetic progestins
~ is suppressed by continuous progestins
~ functions as a mild antidepressant
~ is safe, unlike synthetic progestins,
which have a wide variety of side effects
can be beneficial when applied transdermally
~ can be used to counter the side effects
of synthetic progestins used in contraceptives

Progesterone has been prescribed for:
amenorrhea
dysmenorrhea
endometriosis
functional uterine bleeding
premenstrual tension
threatened or habitual abortion

The following synthetic progestins are among
those in use:
Delalutin...... hydroxyprogesterone
caproate in oil
Provera....... methoxyprogesterone
acetate
Norlutin....... norethindrone
Primolut N... norethisterone
Microlut....... levonorgestrel
Microval...... levonorgestrel

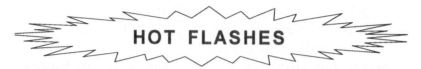

HOT FLASHES

➢ Osteoporosis may be, in part, a progesterone-deficiency disease.
Endocrine Reveiws, 1990[14]
➢ Prescriptions for medroxyprogesterone (synthetic progestin) increased from 2.3 million in 1982 to 11.3 million in 1992, despite cautions.
Obstetrics and Gynecology, 1995[15]
➢ Progesterone alone may be a valuable agent for management of postmenopausal osteoporosis.
Jnl of Bone and Mineral Research, 1990[16]
➢ Progesterone influences skeletal metabolism by promoting bone formation and bone turnover.
Jnl of Obstetrics and Gynecology, 1992[17]
Endocrine Reviews, 1990[18]
➢ Progesterone meets the necessary criteria to play a causal role in mineral metabolism.
Endocrine Reviews, 1990[19]
➢ Postmenopausal women with benign and malignant ovarian tumors have low progesterone levels prior to surgery.
Acta Endocrinologica, 1992[20]

UPDATES
Maturitas 1997 Mar;26(2):103-11
Treatment of urogenital symptoms in postmenopausal women with vaginal progesterone suppositories is shown to be an effective and safe method.

Baillieres Clin Obstet Gynaecol 1996 Sep;10(3):515-30
HRT: the major potential side-effect discussed is ovarian cancer. Non-oral delivery systems for progestins which minimize side-effects will be introduced during the next decade

～～ ENDNOTES ～～ *The fantasy continues...*

Intrigued, we can see that when fatty fish, eggs, butter, and liver are ingested, calcium absorption is more efficient. *Not so with sodas, unleavened bread, milk, or chlorinated water.*

Cow's milk contains four times more calcium than human milk, and so we watch, perplexed, as the breast-fed baby absorbs more calcium than the child who is fed cow's milk! We are amazed when the oxalic acid in spinach, Swiss chard, beet greens, and parsley casts a spell over calcium, rendering it less absorbable.

If the experts cannot sort it out, how can we?

Hormone replacement therapy is not the only area of serious controversy when it comes to the accepted methods of dealing with osteoporosis. Misinformation surrounding calcium absorption and supplementation runs a close second.

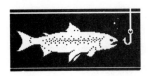

Helps calcium
absorption!

Hinders calcium
absorption!

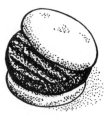

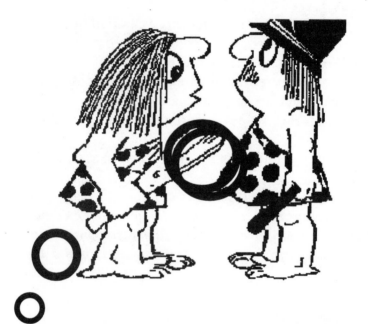

I just invented the wheel. But I know that a few centuries from now, you men will take all the credit.

10

WHAT ABOUT CALCIUM SUPPLEMENTS?

WHY CALCIUM SUPPLEMENTS ARE NOT ENOUGH

If calcium loss is a major part of the problem and we can't get the proper calcium absorption from our modern-day diets, does it make sense to eat more calcium in supplemental form?

> Consider dietary calcium from an evolutionary perspective: *Researchers tell us that the prevailing calcium intake during most of human evolution was substantially higher than it is today.*[1] (No surprises here.)

Taking supplemental calcium in the form of tablets or capsules appears to be an obvious course of action to help guard against osteoporosis. But for reasons that are still not entirely clear, calcium supplementation alone for the purpose of improving bone integrity has been largely ineffective. Let's explore what we know in this area.

An editorial in *New England Journal of Medicine* summarizes the situation:

> *For the past ten years, both scientists and the lay public have been subjected to a spate of claims and counterclaims about the value of ensuring an adequate intake of calcium throughout life. Although the role of calcium supplements in the health of adult bone has been called controversial, it may be more accurate to say that it has been confusing. A recent review identified 43 studies published since 1988 that relate calcium intake to bone mass, bone loss, or bone fragility. Twenty-six reported that calcium intake is associated in some way with bone mass, bone loss, or fracture; 16 do not. In a presidential election, such a majority would be considered a landslide, but for scientists, the 16 negative studies leave a nagging doubt. Does that difference mean that calcium is less important, or perhaps not important at all?[2]*

A report in *Lancet* states that there is no convincing evidence that high calcium intake substantially affects bone loss.[3] *New England Journal of Medicine* reports that no published study sheds useful light on the question of *how much* calcium is needed for bone health.[4] The *Southern Medical Journal* advises that increased calcium intake in supplemental form will *not* increase skeletal mass in mature, premenopausal women, nor will it prevent bone loss in postmenopausal women.[5] *Bone and Mineral* concludes that because iron, zinc and magnesium intake are positively correlated with forearm bone mass content in premenopausal women, *bone mass is influenced by dietary factors other than calcium.*[6]

Another important finding is that calcium *by itself* somehow interferes with vitamin D in its hormonal form. Henry DeLuca MD, known for his research on vitamin D, writes:

> *The emphasis on calcium has taken the focus away from the complexity of the issue and is preventing some kinds of therapy. For example, treatment with the hormonal form of vitamin D cannot be administered with high intakes of calcium.*

> *We tear down our skeleton and build it back about once every five years. If you take large amounts of calcium, you turn off the production of the hormone. That interferes with bone remodeling.*

> *I believe it is okay to take extra calcium, but I don't think anyone should be misled into believing that if she or he has osteoporosis, taking calcium is going to help or cure.*[7]

Two warnings come to mind:

(1) If you have seen references to (or your physician tells you about) studies extolling the benefits of 1,500 milligrams of supplemental calcium per day, take heed. A careful researcher will note that these studies are often not conducted long enough for valid results; that increased bone density may be within the range of error of the testing machines; and that women tested may still be losing bone (as was the case in one popular study). *The loss demonstrated is simply less than losses compared with other women.* Again, we need to be aware of the parameters used as guidelines. Results are rarely compared with natural remedies.

(2) Don't throw the baby out with the bath water. Calcium supplementation has other advantages—significant bone preservation during menopausal years just doesn't happen to be one of them (unless you are truly calcium deficient). Note, too, that many studies are not done with a sharp enough pencil. *Certain forms of calcium, combined with other specific nutrients, produce different results.* For example, supplemental calcium taken with vitamin D$_3$ reduces nonvertebral fractures.[8] And hydrochloric acid is as necessary as vitamin D for healthy bones. For efficient absorption, calcium supplementation MUST be taken with synergistic nutrients.

FIGURE 15

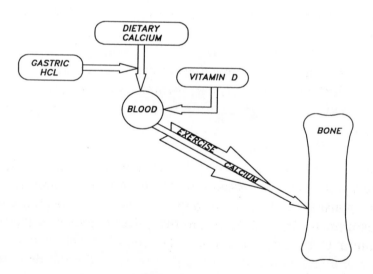

CALCIUM ABSORPTION HELPERS

Gastric hydrochloric acid (HCL) helps the absorption of dietary calcium; hormonal vitamin D is necessary to incorporate calcium into bone structure; and the bone-building process is greatly accelerated by exercise.

Even injecting calcium directly into the bloodstream has little effect on bone health.[9]

The amount of available calcium—dietary or in blood—is not the limiting factor in your ability to maintain the integrity of your bones. (See Figure 15 on page 128.)

When areas of the world with notably low dietary calcium (the South African Bantu region, Hong Kong, and Singapore) are compared with high calcium populations (Britain, Sweden, and the United States), it becomes obvious that high calcium intake alone is not associated with long-lasting healthy bones.[10]

A large number of calcium supplements are available, but many are marketed without proper knowledge of the bioavailability of the actual preparation.[11] This promotes varied conclusions and leads to controversy.

Studies published in *Lancet* show that we have vitamin D receptors which are linked with bone density. Variability of responses may be related to the function of these receptor sites *and* to differences in environmental factors such as vitamin D or calcium content in foods.[12]

Clearly, there are factors at work for bone health other than calcium, and there is still a lot to be learned. But much information is already available. Those of us who have examined the research and clinical results have at least an inkling of what does make a difference. The good news is that many of these factors are easily within our control.

Despite the controversy concerning calcium supplements, most practitioners suggest its use. But absorption varies, since it is dependent on vitamin D intake, exercise, and a host of additional factors, known and unknown. Until more is understood, many practitioners attempt to insure nutritional status by recommending 800 to 1,200 milligrams daily. One gets the impression that it is being prescribed as a safeguard "just in case." (You're not superstitious, but you don't walk under a ladder.)

The RDA for calcium is 800 milligrams for men and women and 1200 for postmenopausal women. If you decide to continue calcium supplementation and increase the dosage to 1200 or 1500 milligrams, magnesium supplementation must be included, along with other important nutrients. Keep in mind that calcium also reduces zinc.

A typical good bone formula contains calcium in the hydroxyapatite and/or calcium citrate or aspartate forms, preferably in low doses. Although bone meal and dolomite are good natural calcium and magnesium sources, contamination with lead and other toxins may be a problem.

In addition to calcium, magnesium, and zinc, well-appointed formulas should contain vitamin D_3, boron, silicon, and even a few vitamins such as beta-carotene, A, K, and folic acid. Shark chondroitin (shark cartilage) is also a good addition because it strengthens and maintains cartilage integrity. Remember that vitamin D and extra hydrochloric acid help to increase the absorption of the calcium supplement.

Yet another beneficial supplement is bovine collagen, backed by excellent medical studies, brand-named *Arthred*.

Calcium with magnesium is a good tranquilizer, so taking this supplement at night is often recommended.

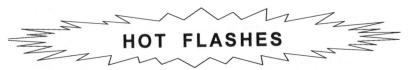

HOT FLASHES

➤ The usefulness of calcium supplementation for the entire population appears to be questionable.
New England Jnl of Medicine, 1995.[13]

➤ Calcium supplementation alone is of little value and is inconsistent with available studies.
Medical Hypotheses, 1988[14]

➤ Substantial bone loss occurs in women despite intake of 750 milligrams of calcium daily.
New England Jnl of Medicine, 1993[15]

➤ Little evidence supports the effectiveness of calcium as a strategy to prevent hip fractures.
Lancet, 1993[16]
New England Jnl of Medicine, 1995[17]

➤ Large intakes of dietary calcium can cause constipation.
Annual Review of Nutrition, 1990[18]

➤ Japanese have lower bone density and lower calcium intake, but have far less fractures than we do.
Proceedings of the Society for Experimental Biology and Medicine, 1992[19]

➤ Other studies demonstrating similar results are widely published in many prestigious journals.[20,21,22,23]

UPDATES

Calcif Tissue International 1997 Jan;60(1):119-23
Activated vitamin D administration is able to reduce bone resorption in postmenopausal, osteoporotic patients with a vitamin D-sufficient status.

American Jnl of Clinical Nutrition 1996 Jun;63(6):950-3
Some studies in adults have shown that high calcium intake may negatively affect magnesium utilization.

American Jnl of Clinical Nutrition 1997 Jun;65(6):1803-9
High-calcium diets can reduce net zinc absorption and balance, increasing zinc requirements.

American Jnl Epidemiol 1997 May 15;145(10):926-34
Calcium supplements were associated with increased
risk of hip and vertebal fractures. No substantial beneficial effect of calcium on fracture risk was found.

Orthopedic Nursing 1996 May-June;15(3):67-71
Women in northern climates are more susceptible to
osteoporosis due to their lack of exposure to sunlight,
which ultimately leads to vitamin D deficiencies.

American Jnl of Medical Science 1996 Dec;312(6):278-86
Treatment of vitamin D deficiency is associated with
significant reductions in the number of hip fractures.

NOTES ON CALCIUM IN FOODS

Two large dried figs contain 80 mgs of calcium.
But it takes 156 saltine crackers to get the same
80 mgs. One portion of raw green vegetables
offers 250 mgs of calcium; 4 ounces of salmon,
291 mgs. Summer vegetables have more calcium
than fall or winter vegetables.

Calcium absorption is decreased by cocoa, bran,
wheat germ, phosphorus foods (meat, cheese,
and soda pop), and oxalic acid foods (beet greens,
chard, spinach, rhubarb). High protein diets are
also calcium-depleting.

Additional calcium antagonists are chlorine (as
in tap water—see page 144), and drugs including
cortisone, antacids, laxatives, and diuretics.

Butterfat promotes the absorption of calcium. The
fat content of one or two or even three glasses
of whole milk daily, as compared with skim or
low-fat, will not affect weight or cholesterol levels,
as advertisements suggest. (The major cholesterol
culprits are *processed* fats and stress.)

~~ ENDNOTES ~~ *The fantasy continues...*

My fantasy transports us to Brazil's southeastern Atlantic forest, where we study the menu of a monkey— the *muriquis*. This primate self-medicates. The purpose of our junket is to see *how* and try to discern *why*.

We note that from late September to mid-October, when banquets of edible fruit abound, the muriquis monkeys eat mainly the leaves of only two plants of the legume family. The monkeys actually camp out at the leaf sources, behaving as if these leaves were the most delectable of all fruits. (They are not.) And then they seek another fruit, known as *monkey ear*. But here they take only small nibbles, as we might do when sampling a strange hors d'oeuvre at a cocktail party.

Ordinarily, the muriquis prefer more succulent fruits, even if it takes a greater effort to locate them. So why the change in preference at this time of year? By eating the leguminous leaves instead of the fruits, both male and female appear to get a surge of protein, *which fortifies them for the upcoming mating season.*

But why the monkey ear fruit? Guess what! Monkey ear contains *stigmasterol*, a steroid used in the laboratory for the manufacture of progesterone! Recent studies indicate that plant hormones can regulate reproduction in some animals. It is suggested that stigmasterol is linked to the monkeys' seasonal fertility.[24]

Since we can dream anything, let's assume we have viewed the cellular structure of the foods consumed by the muriqui. Then let us bring this information to our own bodies to have more insight into what it is we should be eating— and how *we, too,* can safely self-medicate.

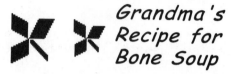 **Grandma's Recipe for Bone Soup**

Veal joints (knuckles) or young chicken bones, or beef neck , or any young cancellous (latticelike) bones

1 cup barley
2 to 3 quarts water
green vegetables in season
(the more the better)
seasonings to taste

Cook bones and barley in water. Bring to boil and simmer over low heat ½ hour.

Nutrition Tip: No better soup for your aching bones!

11

FOOD AS SELF-MEDICATION

FEMALE AND FEELING FINE

There are easy measures you can take to keep your bones healthy and your hormones flowing properly. Best of all, these practices help to prevent discomfort. You should also understand that although discomfort is typical, it is definitely not normal.

Some of these steps are easy, but others may tax your powers of self-discipline to the limit. No two individuals respond exactly the same way, and any of these suggestions could be critical for you. Keep in mind that, unlike drugs, natural procedures for improving health don't always work instantly. You didn't lose bone density in a day. So give nature a little time here. Young or old, *you can turn things around!*

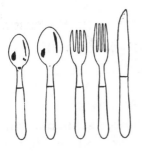

What you put in your mouth every day of your life affects the length and quality of your entire life.

Eat Your Vegetables

Eat your veggies! Timeless, simple advice. Green leafy vegetables are your best source of calcium. Far better than milk, it turns out.

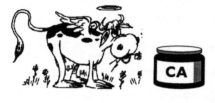

Where does all that calcium in milk come from, anyway? Do you see the farmer giving calcium pills to the cows?

This is a key element of any successful program for reversing osteoporosis. Perhaps veggies work as a good source of calcium because of the cofactor nutrients they contain—silicon, boron, beta-carotene, and even vitamin C. Vegetables are also a more direct source of calcium: The cow eats the stuff that grows in the ground, makes the milk, and you drink the milk. Why not eat the food that grows in the ground to begin with? Maybe it's like taping a video from another video, rather than buying the original. Each copy "loses a generation," reducing quality. An oversimplification, but you get the point.

Avoid Dairy Products

Once upon a time, avoiding dairy products flew in the face of conventional wisdom. But it's *de rigeur* now!

> **Cow's milk is a perfect food—for a calf!**

Humans were never designed to drink cow's milk. With such an abundance of healthful food choices available, milk should be considered as a slightly more subtle kind of junk food, to be avoided or used in limited quantities. Low-fat and nonfat milk are even worse.

> The fat in milk plays an important role in the digestion and assimilation of its other nutrients—*including calcium!* Drinking low-fat or no-fat milk is not in your best bone-health interest.

A very high percentage of North Americans are lactose-intolerant to some degree and should avoid milk for health reasons. Casein (the protein in milk) binds minerals. *Because of its high level of animal protein, milk consumption may cause greater calcium loss than gain.*[1] Note: Half the diabetics in this country are milk-sensitive.

Homogenization makes the situation worse. Particles of milk fat are reduced in size and increased in number, causing more surface area for detrimental action. The faster absorption rate of these tiny fat particles can be a problem. Unhomogenized milk is hard to find, but it is superior; or, more accurately, less damaging.

As stated earlier, there's also the danger that milk may add dietary estrogen and other hormones—now used freely in animals by the dairy industry. True, first-pass liver treatment attempts to remove these foreign hormones, but, as discussed, there is uncertainty as to how much of the unwanted constituents are ignored by your liver.

Fermented products with viable culture, such as the yogurt produced by nutrition-aware companies (available in health stores and an occasional supermarket), may be a more acceptable alternative. Lactase (the lactose- or milk-metabolizing enzyme) is produced in the fermentation process, so fermented milk products are often tolerated by the milk-sensitive, even though these foods are milk-based.

> Try plain yogurt as a milk substitute on breakfast cereal. Substitute watered-down yogurt in recipes when milk is called for.

Avoid Junk Foods

You already know that you should avoid junk foods. Easier said than done, isn't it? Like many Americans, you may feel guilty when you consume such food, but not guilty enough to abstain.

Does it surprise you that sugar affects your bones? If you are concerned about osteoporosis, perhaps you will be a little more selective when making food choices if you know that sugar increases calcium excretion.

Complete dentures are required by 44 percent of osteoporotic patients before the age of 60, compared with only 15 percent of non-osteoporotics. Mandibular bone density shows significant correlations with bone density elsewhere, particularly in the hip. Dentists are in a unique position to diagnose osteoporosis prior to the loss of a debilitating amount of bone, as reported in *Lancet*, 1995. This risk factor needs greater attention.

The teeth of osteoporotics don't degrade along with bones. Teeth are built differently; they don't lose calcium or accept it the way healthy bones do. But there are connections.

> The same dietary factors that destroy teeth also take their toll on the rest of your body, and that includes sugar consumption.

Avoid Junk Drinks

What's a junk drink? Almost every beverage except pure spring water.

Milk

We've already discussed milk, and although this may be hard to accept, I have to classify cow's milk as a junk drink.

Sodas

Sodas are devastating to bone health because of their phosphorus content. When physicians study results of bone photon tests, they can actually identify the 18- and 19-year-olds who drink the colas.

Coffee

Coffee is dangerous because of its effect on pH balance. Dr. Corsello explains:

> *A good natural defense against osteoporosis is to keep the acidity of your blood in proper balance. If you don't, your body will, by removing calcium from your bones to defend the pH balance in your blood.*"[2]

An interesting point! Also note that smoking and alcohol, in addition to coffee, raise blood acidity. Coffee is a tough one because it is firmly entrenched in daily routines, if not in our culture—to say nothing of its mild addictive quality. My personal conclusion is that coffee and soft drinks contribute to more osteoporosis than current thinking acknowledges. I'm not waiting for more research. These drinks are out of my diet permanently.

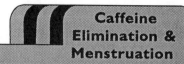
CAFFEINE ELIMINATION

ABSTRACT: The rate at which caffeine is eliminated from your body decreases as the levels of sex steroids increase. Pregnancy or intake of oral contraceptives are among the reasons for increasing sex steroids. [This may be why so many women can't drink coffee when pregnant—the nausea that ensues because of slow removal could be nature's protection against increased caffeine intake at a critical time.]

Changes in sex steroid levels that occur during normal menstrual cycling may also affect the rate of caffeine elimination. Evidence suggests that elimination may be slowed in the late luteal phase, prior to the onset of menstruation. Such a reduction leads to increased accumulation of caffeine in the face of repeated intake during the day.

Lane JD; Steege JF; Rupp SL; Kuhn CM. Menstrual cycle effects on caffeine elimination in the human female. *European Journal of Clinical Pharmacology*, 1992, 43(5):543-6.

Fruit Juice

Fruit drinks (even those that have no sugar added) are too sweet—too high in simple carbohydrates—to be nutritionally valuable. Note the metabolic differences that occur when you consume apple juice compared with eating whole apples containing the same number of calories:

After apple juice
- ➤ Insulin responses are 50 percent greater
- ➤ You are hungry sooner
- ➤ Your cholesterol levels are higher
- ➤ A rebound fall in glucose follows

Ready-to-drink fruit juices may also have more fluoride than your body can handle comfortably. (See pages 143 and 156 for more information on fluoride.) The source, of course, is the water added to fruit concentrates.[3]

Hard to accept, isn't it, considering how long fruit juices have been promoted as healthful and "natural." To make powdered and granulated supplements more palatable, try adding only about an inch of pure fruit juice to filtered water. You may find this small amount of juice just as helpful for making the mix acceptable as when you use a full glass of fruit juice. (Another hint for making mixes more tasteful is the use of beet crystals. See page 180.)

When it comes to fruit juice, the low end of moderation is good, but abstinence is best. Try to eat the whole fruit instead—it really is more satisfying. (If you must drink juices, avoid those that are packaged in aluminum cans. Glass containers are preferable, especially for tomato juice. The acid in tomato juice is a great magnet for metals.)

What About Other Liquids?

Fresh vegetable juices are another story. They can have tremendous therapeutic value, and if you're lucky enough to have a good juicer, there are times you want to put it to use.

> Most vegetables contain good ratios of calcium and phosphorus. Some even have more calcium than phosphorus. (The latter include alfalfa, parsley, dandelion greens, and chard, to name a few.)

Because the concentration of minerals in the American diet is not high, large quantities of vegetables should be consumed to compensate for the offenses of our real-world diets. Juicing vegetables can help.

Cautions are necessary here, too. Vegetable juice degenerates nutritionally with incredible speed —it's been claimed that the "half-life" of a glass of carrot juice is only 12 minutes. Additional problems: carrot juice kept at room temperature for 24 hours has unfavorable concentrations of carcinogenic nitrites.[4]

And isn't juice itself unnatural? How can we justify drinking a liquid that contains 10 or 20 times the amount of constituents than would be found in the unprocessed vegetables? And what about the fiber that gets lost in the juicing process? These are valid concerns, and that's why I eat most of my vegetables whole. Vegetable juices can be *therapeutic*; whole vegetables can be *preventive*. Our vegetable juicer comes to life at the first sign of any health problem. Otherwise it remains dormant.

So we're left with water. Oh, did I mention fluoridation? Fluoride therapy was once considered potentially beneficial for the treatment of osteoporosis because it increases bone mass. Fluoride, however, is destructive to connective tissue, causing a wide assortment of ligament, tendon, periarticular (situated around a joint), and bone problems.[5]

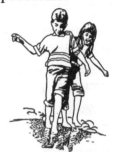

"I'm getting thirsty.
What kind of bottled water
do your parents buy?"

Fluoride may increase *bone mass*, but it does nothing to increase bone *strength*. Think of an old concrete bridge, with the concrete dry and brittle. You can make the roadway thicker by adding a layer of gravel to the surface. Now you have more mass and more material. But have you made the bridge any stronger?

Nonvertebral fractures increase 300 to 600 percent in patients undergoing fluoride therapy.[6]

Extensive research shows that even a *low* level of fluoridation correlates with higher fracture statistics.[7,8,9]

A report in the *Journal of the American Medical Association* showed a significant increase in hip fractures in men and women over 65 in Brigham City, Utah, where the water is fluoridated at 1 part per million (the assumed safe level) when compared with two other cities in Utah which have only 0.3 parts per million.

This is one of many examples of links between fluoridated water and extended incidents of hip fractures published in the last few years.[10]

Based on all this information, if you live in a city where fluoridation is in use, you should take tap water off the list, too. There's still controversy, unfortunately, about whether fluoridation is a useful strategy for improving the dental health of children. The gap in the tooth decay rate in children living in fluoridated and nonfluoridated water districts has been narrowing. Studies have found that the divergence has all but disappeared.[11] An article in *Chemical and Engineering News*, April 1994, reported that a "dental screening of 26,000 elementary school children showed that the more fluoride a child drank, the more cavities appeared in the teeth."

> **Note that no health benefits are claimed for older adults with fluoridated water, and a consensus is developing that fluoridation can be harmful to the mature population.**

I have never allowed my family to consume fluoridated water when I could control the situation.

One more problem concerning water: *Chlorinated water, especially if consumed on a high fat diet, reduces calcium absorption.*[12] Almost all tap water is chlorinated. If the kitchen faucet MUST be your water source, fill a pitcher with water and let it stand uncovered, either in the fridge or at room temperature, for 24 hours. Most of the chlorine will evaporate.[13]

Are you concluding that perils lurk at every swallow? How about spring water, perhaps with a twist of lemon or lime to embellish your drink? In most cities you can have good water delivered (like milk in the old days).

Cut Down on Meat

You've heard it again and again, but little attention is paid to this fact: Too much protein causes calcium to be lost in the urine. How much protein do you need? That depends on the *quality* of the protein you are consuming. As a general rule, the requirement is for no more than one and one-half ounces of protein for a 150-pound person per day. That's not a lot, is it? It translates to very little meat or cheese. And even that specified amount is arbitrary.

FIGURE 16

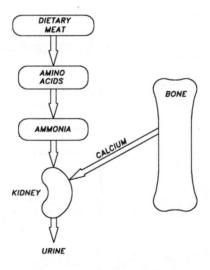

MEAT CONSUMPTION
AND CALCIUM EXCRETION

Amino acid metabolism that results from meat consumption causes calcium to be pulled out of bone tissue.

> Things get worse as we get older, but we can exert a certain amount of control. For example, senior meat eaters lose almost twice as much calcium as their vegetarian peers—a demonstration of how we control our own longevity destiny!

A meat-eating animal in the wild balances its calcium deficiency and phosphorus excess by consuming bones. Any veterinarian will confirm that when dogs are fed leftover hamburger or commercially-prepared all-meat dog food, skeletal disease is the consequence.

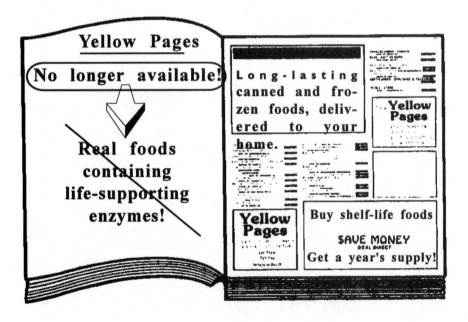

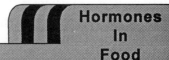

MEMOS — Hormones In Food

HORMONES IN FOOD

ABSTRACT In the absence of effective federal regulation, the meat industry uses hundreds of animal-feed additives, including antibiotics, tranquilizers, pesticides, animal drugs, artificial flavors, industrial wastes, and *growth-promoting hormones*, with little or no concern about the carcinogenic and other toxic effects of dietary residues of these additives. Illustratively, after decades of misleading assurances of the safety of diethylstilbestrol (DES) and its use as a growth-promoting animal-feed additive, the United States finally banned its use in 1979, some 40 years after it was first shown to be carcinogenic. The meat industry then promptly switched to other carcinogenic additives, particularly the sex hormones estradiol, progesterone, and testosterone, which are implanted in the ears of more than 90 percent of commercially raised feedlot cattle. Unlike the synthetic DES, residues of which can be monitored and use of which was conditional on a seven-day preslaughter withdrawal period, residues of hormones are not detectable, since they cannot be practically differentiated from the same hormones produced by the body. The relationship between recently increasing cancer rates and the lifetime exposure of the U.S. population to dietary residues of these and other unlabeled carcinogenic feed additives is a matter of critical public health concern.

Epstein SS. The chemical jungle: today's beef industry.
International Journal of Health Services, 1990, 20(2):277-80.

Reduce Phosphorus Intake

Recall that phosphorus is an integral part of bone material but that ingesting too much is not in your best health interest. It's the *proportion* of phosphorus to calcium that's significant. In the presence of too much phosphorus, hormonal feedback mechanisms can block the proper assimilation of phosphorus *and* calcium.[14] The average American diet, high in phosphorus, just doesn't offer the recommended one-to-one calcium/phosphorus ratio.

So even though cheese (unlike meat) contains high amounts of calcium, the calcium is no match for the phosphorus content. Consuming high calcium foods like milk doesn't serve to correct the problem or alter the ratio. Here's one reason why: Milk and milk products are almost equal sources of both phosphorus and calcium but sometimes contain even more phosphorus. (Cottage cheese is an example—it has considerably more phosphorus than calcium.) At higher levels of ingestion, calcium absorption decreases sharply. You are an efficient calcium picker-upper only when calcium is present at low levels.

> Even if the same quantities of calcium and phosphorus are consumed (as in milk and milk products), the absorption ratio shifts so that more phosphorus than calcium gets absorbed—thereby disturbing the health-promoting ratio.

At the risk of repetition, please check Table 4 on the next page for a list of phosphorus-loaded foods.

TABLE 4
HIGH PHOSPHORUS FOODS

➤ Almost all processed and canned meats (hot dogs, ham, bacon)
➤ Processed cheeses
➤ Baked products that include phosphate baking powder (commonly used)
➤ Cola and other soft drinks
➤ Instant soups and puddings
➤ Toppings and seasonings
➤ Breads
➤ Cereals
➤ Meats (meat contains *fifty times* more phosphorus than calcium!)
➤ Potatoes
➤ Phosphate food additives: phosphoric acid; pyrophosphate; polyphosphates (including chelators), sequestering and emulsifying agents, acidulators, water binders (including sodium phosphate, potassium phosphate, and phosphoric acid).

Quite a list, and too bad; it includes foods that I personally don't want to give up (baked potatoes, for example).

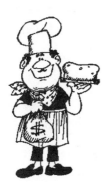

The more processed, the higher the profits.

Charts can help you evaluate the phosphorus and calcium content of many popular foods. There are surprises here, too; not all healthful foods are high in calcium, and some have copious amounts of phosphorus! Use the data as a rough guide to gauge your *average* calcium/phosphorus ratio, but don't make a religion of avoiding unprocessed high-phosphorus foods. Those that have not been commercially mushed, mashed, or mangled have other nutritional redeeming features. Soft drinks have none. Real foods—such as whole grains and potatoes—do.

Avoid Harmful Packaging

High levels of tin may be found in some processed foods due to the addition of tin-based preservatives and stabilizers, or to corrosion and leaching of the metal from unlacquered cans, and even from tin foils used in packaging. Diets comprised of high proportions of canned vegetables and canned fish could supply amounts of tin in excess of acceptable quantities. Phosphate food additives: phosphoric acid; pyrophosphate; polyphosphates (including chelators), sequestering and emulsifying agents, acidulators, water binders (including sodium phosphate, potassium phosphate, and phosphoric acid). A variety of adverse effects with the use of tin have been reported, including those on the calcium content of bone.[15]

Worse, the linings of some brands of canned peas emit synthetic estrogens devastatingly more powerful than the estrogen you manufacture in your body.

Packaging and labels can be deceiving. Shop wisely.

Avoid Aluminum in Underarm Spray and in Antacids

Environmental exposure to aluminum is increasing universally. Aluminum is commonly found in food, medicine, and cosmetics. Sources include antacids, underarm sprays, cookware (especially when used to prepare acid foods such as tomato sauce), air conditioning (sorry about that), environmental contamination, children's aspirin, some baking powders, many white flours, and foods grown in toxic soil.

Aluminum from antacids has become a serious problem because it has been shown to be absorbed twenty to thirty times more than would occur with aluminum from other sources.[16] Aluminum poisoning and spontaneous fractures are definite associations. Aluminum-induced bone problems may be more widespread than we previously realized.

You can be more selective. Purchase unleaded cans of food; look for aluminum-free sprays and baking powder; and use stainless steel, enamel, or glass cookware. Aluminum-free digestive aids are available.

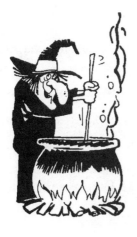

I wonder why I got that subpoena from the FDA demanding to know what additives I use.

Grow Your Own Sprouts

Grow your own sprouts, or at least buy them and eat them. Sprouts are a good source of absorbable calcium and they are low in phosphorus. They are likely to be your only source of fresh food—growing up to the moment they enter your mouth—a dim reflection of an era when all food was that fresh, and very important for many reasons that don't directly concern us here.

Suffice it to say that you're doing yourself a great disservice if you don't buy or grow sprouts. Seeds may be consumed at any stage of sprouting, but harvesting at peak offers the most value. Vitamin C is actually synthesized during germination. The concentrations of some of the B vitamins are also increased, along with other nutrients. Since seeds vary, it's advisable to experiment, using a good book on sprouting as a starting guide.

Alfalfa, mung, and chickpeas are excellent sprouts for beginners. I purchase already-sprouted sunflower seeds (called sunflower lettuce) and buckwheat. I sprout my own clover, radish, lentil, chickpeas, green peas, wheatberries, mung, azuki, barley, and alfalfa. (Recall that alfalfa is a phytoestrogen.)

Exercise—Outdoors

There is no controversy when we discuss exercise and the need for natural outdoor exposure. Everyone agrees that moderate weight-bearing movement stimulates bones to keep them strong.

Bookstores are full of publications about aerobic programs written by people with far more expertise in this area. If you don't already have a reasonable exercise plan, walk to the nearest bookstore—leave your car where it is.

I'll add one note, though. Fast walking is still the best exercise around. It's safe, weight-bearing, relatively low-impact, always available, absolutely free, and you already know how to do it. (As Dr. Lee says, "Walking is good for the bowels, good for circulation, and good for seeing what the neighbors are doing.")

If you want additional back-strengthening strategies, go dancing or check out some of the exercise machines. Excessive activity, however, can inhibit bone growth and gives rise to stress fractures.[17] One reason is the loss of calcium that occurs during vigorous exercise. Other nutrients are lost with exercise overindulgence, too.

When you are a seasoned walker, try experimenting with a few different types of motion. Pretend you are the Tin Man in *The Wizard of Oz*. You will walk with muscles more tense and this will slow you down. Then see yourself as a rag doll, with your whole body loose, arms swinging freely, taking larger strides. This Raggedy Anne mode is far better.

If you are right-handed, the bones on your left side are more apt to break than those on your right side.[18] This demonstrates that exercised bones are less subject to damage. A routine of physical activity may be as beneficial for your skeleton as it is for your heart.

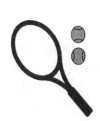

A daily exercise program can make a significant difference in every phase of your health.

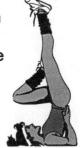

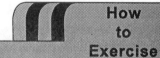

MEMOS

How to Exercise

WHY WALKING IS BEST

In addition to its beneficial effects on bone, exercise stimulates hormonal secretions and may create euphoria more powerful than mood-elevating drugs. Osteoporosis is a nutrition-deficiency disease. The right kind of exercise is an important component of nutrition.

Good exercise is both aerobic and weight-bearing. Aerobic exercises are those that make your heart accelerate for a sustained period of time, causing a need for more air (oxygen). An aerobic exercise is go-go-go and not stop-and-go. Weight-bearing exercises keep you on your feet. Tennis and golf are weight-bearing, but not aerobic. Swimming is aerobic, but not weight-bearing. Fast walking is the best possible exercise.

An exercise session should last for at least twenty minutes. If optimal benefit is the goal, plan to do your aerobic activity at least five times a week.

Regular outdoor walking schedules guarantee that both your body and eyes will be exposed to daylight. This causes increased output of various glandular secretions and promotes absorption of priceless vitamin D, the power substance for the prevention of osteoporosis.

No matter how old you are or what level of activity you participated in before starting, fitness can be achieved with continuous vigorous walking for regular periods of time each day. (You see, there are no excuses.)

If you think you have no time for walking, the good news is that the energy bonus helps you to get that time back!

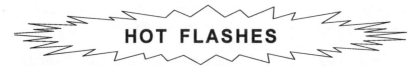

HOT FLASHES

➤ As caffeine intake increases, so does the risk of hip fracture.

New England Jnl of Medicine, 1995[19]

➤ Caffeine (from coffee, tea, and/or soda) stimulates the release of calcium from bone.

Calcified Tissue International, 1992[20]

➤ The vegetarian diet has a higher nutrient density for folate, thiamin, vitamin C, and vitamin A. It also contains less total fat, saturated fatty acids, and cholesterol, plus higher dietary fiber.

American Jnl of Clinical Nutrition, 1988[21]

➤ Hip fracture risk decreases as the distance walked per day increases.

New England Jnl of Medicine, 1995[22]

➤ Those who follow a vegetarian diet for at least 20 years have about an 18 percent bone mineral loss by age 80, whereas meat eaters have 35 percent less bone mineral at that age.

American Jnl of Clinical Nutrition, 1988[23]

➤ Although there is a gain in bone density from fluoride ingestion, fluoride increases fracture risk.

Revue du Rhumatisme et des Maladies Osteo-Articulaires, 1992[24]

➤ Sodium fluoride cannot be recommended for routine use at this time.

PostGraduate Medicine, 1990[25]

➤ Preservation of bone mass through early premenopausal life can be favored by *good nutrition and physical activity*.

Clinical Rheumatology, 1989
Osteoporosis International, 1990[26,27]

➤ Women on oral contraceptives are more susceptible to osteoporosis in later years because of diminished levels of magnesium.

American Jnl of Clinical Nutrition, 1964[28]

➢ Athletic women become amenorrheic if *undernutrition* coexists with increasing exercise loads.
Sports Medicine, 1992[29]

➢ Milk and milk products are among the poorest sources of copper—a mineral protective against osteoporosis. Lactose, as in dairy products, may interfere with copper metabolism.
Medical Hypotheses, 1988[30]

➢ An exercise/hormone regimen is more effective than exercise and calcium supplementation for increasing bone mass.
New England Jnl of Medicine, 1991[31]

➢ Current smokers have about twice as high a risk of hip fracture as nonsmokers or former smokers.
New England Jnl of Medicine, 1995[32]

UPDATES

Molecular Cellular Biochem 1997 Mar;168(1-2):117-23
Flax-seed has shown beneficial effects in cancer and lupus nephritis.

Jnl of Bone Mineral Research 1996 Dec;11(12):1905-12
Acute ingestion of phosphate leads to an acute inactivation of the early phase of bone formation. [A good reason to curtail children' s soft drink consumption.]

Osteoporosis International 1996;6(5):361-7
General aerobic exercise may reduce overall fracture risk, even though it doesn't significantly increase bone density.

Bone 1996 Jan;18(1 Suppl):37S-43S
There is increasing evidence that load-bearing is an important, if not the most important, functional influence on bone mass and architecture.

Bone 1996 Dec;19(6):595-601
Fluoridated water caused osteomalacia and reduced bone strength in test animals under certain conditions.

~~ ENDNOTES ~~ The fantasy continues...

Now we view the consequences of the many high-tech foods: ice cream that won't melt, grains grown quickly with artificial fertilizer, peanut butter that doesn't have to be mixed, salt flowing freely, butter that doesn't have to be refrigerated, butter that's yellow all year round, cream in milk that doesn't rise to the top, potato chips never going soggy, bread staying soft, rice that doesn't stick to the pot, rice cooking in a minute, mashed potatoes available in a box, breaded shrimp pieces all the same size, and sweet cream—30 days old—still smelling fresh. Oy! We can even see why tomatoes won't crack when hurled against a wall at 12 miles an hour!

How can we protect ourselves against the toxins used to make these foods so convenient? How can we put back into our food that which should have been there to begin with? Are we ready to take away substances that don't belong there? I believe, along with many researchers and clinical practitioners the world over, that a major part of the answer—until we can turn things around—is the use of supplements.

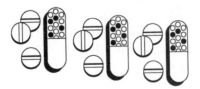

Webster's

sup.ple.ment
(1) something added to complete a thing;
(2) something added to supply a deficiency.

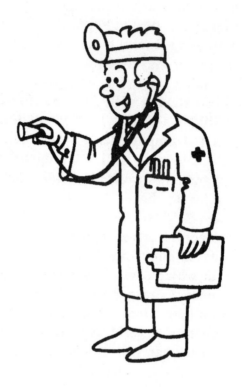

If you continue with quick-fix pudding, instant coffee, jiffy-fast supper and super swift-quick dinners, you can look forward to an early, quick, swift, instant death.

12

SUPPLEMENTS FOR HEALTH

WHY FOOD IS NOT ENOUGH

Take Your Vitamins

Vitamin C

If it had been up to me to name vitamins, I would have named this one first. It's hard to find any disorder for which no improvement is shown with the addition of vitamin C. This nutrient has an incredible number of different metabolic roles.

Vitamin C is a *water-soluble antioxidant*, which means two things:

(1) It protects complicated proteins from oxidation—that is, destruction that occurs by combining with oxygen.

(2) It is easily carried to and from places needed because it dissolves in water.

A report in the *American Journal of Epidemiology* (1996;144:165) showed that women who consume at least 500 milligrams of vitamin C daily are at lower risk for breast cancer.

Among the lesser-known functions of vitamin C is its role in collagen, the flexible part of your composite bone structure.

Vitamin C helps to repair collagen and to build it up. So an ample supply of vitamin C is important for good bone health. We know just a little about how and why.

How much vitamin C should you take? No dosage could be suggested for you without knowledge of your cellular chemistry. Most researchers and physicians agree, however, that the recommended daily allowance of only 60 milligrams is far too scant—either for therapy *or* prevention. That amount is widely acknowledged to be unrealistically low.

At the other end of the scale, Robert Cathcart, MD, of San Mateo, California, has had excellent results with ill patients using therapeutic doses of up to *50 grams*. That's 50,000 milligrams![1] High doses are justified by comparing the amounts of vitamin C synthesized by other mammals who make their own vitamin C. Under stress, these animals increase their production of this nutrient manyfold. On this basis, high doses of vitamin C appear to be reasonable. (It is theorized that humans and a few other animals once had, but eventually lost, this convenient capability.)

Another rationale for taking high doses is that animals manufacture vitamin C in their cells, but we have to swallow it, so some gets lost during digestion.

Overdosing on vitamin C is almost impossible because it's usually easy to determine when you've taken more than you can use. Mild diarrhea or stomach rumbling is the alarm signal—a quick consequence of exceeding the so-called "bowel-tolerance" level. Eating vitamin C to bowel tolerance means increasing your intake by increments of 100, 250, or even 500 milligrams every week or so—until your stomach reacts. Then you back off to the last comfortable dose, and that amount becomes your daily requirement.

> At times of stress or illness, the amount of vitamin C that causes your stomach to scream back at you is significantly higher. You require a lot more vitamin C when you are not up to par, and so your body needs, absorbs, and tolerates more.

Personally, I take about 6 or 7 grams (6,000 to 7,000 milligrams) of vitamin C per day, mostly in an esterified form. I require that amount to keep me free of the respiratory problems I suffered growing up—problems that still plague me whenever I reduce the quantity. I increase the dosage when I am under physical or emotional stress.

Vitamin D

As so clearly explained in the *Journal of Cellular Biochemistry*, the main regulator of calcium absorption is vitamin D. This nutrient is manufactured in your skin under the influence of ultra violet light and is found in limited amounts in only a few foods (egg yolk, certain species of fish, fish liver, and butter). Vitamin D is then converted to more potent forms (or metabolites) in your liver and kidney. With advancing age and skin-cancer scares, men and women tend to have less and less sunlight exposure—the leading natural source of vitamin D.[2]

Among the theories to explain estrogen therapy's effectiveness is one that indicates that estrogen helps the conversion of vitamin D to its active hormonal form—vitamin D_3.

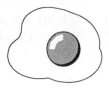

Egg yolks are a good source of vitamin D.

A deficiency of vitamin D is all it takes to develop seriously unhealthy bones. Despite the fact that milk and other foods are routinely fortified with vitamin D, even healthy people are often found to be vitamin-D deficient.

The best insurance against vitamin D deficiency is to spend more time in the sunlight, where the vitamin D is free! A 30-minute 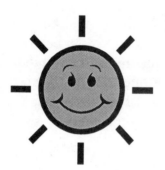 sun-bath should provide 300 to 350 units of vitamin D.[3] An hour is even better, but if time in the sun is not possible, the amount of vitamin D_3 found in a good multivitamin supplement should help to fill the need.

Keep in mind that vitamin D absorption diminishes with age. Lucky are those of us who grew up with Mama insisting we take cod-liver oil. Today, emulsified cod-liver oil is a good supplemental source of vitamin D.

Adequate levels of vitamin D can help prevent osteoporosis in both women *and* men.[4]

When you look at the metabolic pathways involved for vitamin D—from the sun or food to bone formation—you can understand why researchers refer to osteoporosis as a disease of the liver and kidneys! (See Figure 17 on page 163.)

Boron and magnesium, among other minerals, also have roles to play in vitamin D utilization. Perhaps that's why these nutrients are crucial to bone health. (See the sections on these minerals later in this chapter.)

It's important to remember that supplementation with vitamin D reduces bone loss and fracture incidence.

FIGURE 17

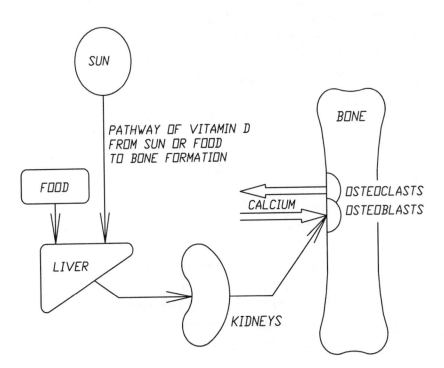

VITAMIN D FROM SOURCE TO BONE

For calcium to be incorporated into your bone structure, vitamin D is a necessity. But this nutrient is provided only by sunlight exposure and by a limited number of foods not commonly consumed.

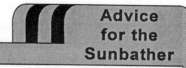

MEMOS

Advice
for the
Sunbather

WORSHIP THE SUN—
JUST A LITTLE

Don't hide in the shade 100 percent of the time because of skin cancer warnings. Skin cancer comes from your body's lack of antioxidants—necessary for coping with overexposure. Limited exposure (up to one hour a day) can improve your health status.

Just don't forget your antioxidants, including:

> - vitamin A
> - beta-carotene
> - vitamin C
> - vitamin E
> - selenium
> - zinc
> - OPCs (proanthocyanidins)
  In the presence of healthy metabolism, these antioxidants help escort toxins right out of your system.

(As my young grandson said when he learned about antioxidants, "Oh, so it's not my A-B-C's I have to pay attention to, but my A-C-E's.")

Vitamin A & Beta-Carotene

Vitamin A is particularly essential for maintaining the integrity of your intestinal walls so they can absorb nutrients (like calcium) with optimal efficiency. Vitamin A and more specifically its precursor, *beta-carotene,* have been shown to provide a measurable protective effect against many types of cancer. While vitamin A itself is fat soluble and can be toxic in extremely high doses, beta-carotene is water soluble and is a much safer nutritional supplement. Nearly every cell can convert beta-carotene to vitamin A as needed—provided your thyroid is in good functioning shape and that you have enough zinc (among other lesser-known relationships).

> **The enzyme that converts beta-carotene to vitamin A uses zinc for the conversion.**

Vitamin A is found in animal foods and beta-carotene is found in ample quantities in yellow and deep green vegetables and fruit. A large raw carrot contains about 11,000 IU (international units). Most nutrition-oriented physicians suggest 25,000 IU per day as a reasonable supplement.[5]

My personal approach is to keep plenty of fresh carrots on hand (organic when available), and these, together with sprouts, are my most frequently-eaten basic snack. I save most of the beta-carotene supplements for the days when I can't eat at least an organic carrot or two along with handfuls of sunflower "lettuce" and/or other green sprouts.

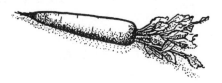

Vitamin E

Vitamin E is often recommended by physicians who specialize in treating women because this nutrient plays a role in the production and metabolism of sex hormones.

> **Vitamin E can enhance the utilization of estrogen stores in your adrenal glands or fat tissues.[6]**

Vitamin E also helps to alleviate breast tenderness. In fact, deficiency of this nutrient is associated with breast cancer. Vitamin E has also been shown to slow the process of skin wrinkling and to protect bone marrow from toxicity.[7,8]

If you are a PMS victim, note that vitamin E is related to the interactions in the multiple biochemical conversions that lead to prostaglandin production. Many of the nutrients that help to alleviate PMS also help to mitigate menopause symptoms, vitamin E among them..

Here's another way to add vitamin E on a daily basis: Soak a tablespoon of wheatberries for 8 to 12 hours; rinse; sprout the seeds for a day or two (rinsing two or three times daily). Your sprouted wheatberries will be sweet and crunchy—great in salads or just as is. You couldn't find a more inexpensive way of getting untampered, fresh wheat germ oil plus fiber. Commercially derived wheat germ oil comes from the germ of the wheatberry, and fiber from its coat.

Sprouted wheatberry seeds are chock full of natural vitamin E and have a high fiber content.

Take Your Minerals

Silicon

Did you know that silicon is the second most abundant element on earth, second only to oxygen? It's as plentiful as sand on the beach—literally! Yet this substance has enormous capacity to turn degenerative processes of aging and disease into regenerative processes of healing and vitality. Silicon is so universal in biological function and so common in our environment that it is taken for granted.

> Despite its abundance, our diets are seriously silicon-deficient.

When food is processed, fiber is usually the first to go, and silicon disappears with it. Stripped cereals and other treated foods have reduced our supplies of this valuable mineral.

Silicon plays its most conspicuous role in calcium metabolism. Mounting evidence points to organic vegetable silicon as one of the key factors in the control of osteoporosis.

It has been conjectured that people in other countries who have no bone disorders despite not getting enough calcium (by our standards) are probably consuming adequate amounts of silicon.[9]

With the exception of mother's milk, silicon levels tend to be higher in plant foods than in foods from animal sources. Foods highest in silicon include grains—especially oats, barley, and the fiber faction of brown rice.[10,11] Silicon is also found in many fruits and vegetables. (See the silicon Food Tables on page 261.)

The herb *equisetum*, commonly known as *horsetail*, is a particularly good source of silicon. Horsetail is a wayside weed that grows nearly everywhere. It's one of those ancient herbs used for millennia. Horsetail tea, for example, has long been recommended for the regeneration of fingernails. I have been an advocate of horsetail extract for decades.

Note that *silicone*, ending with an "e," usually refers to an inorganic form of the mineral which is not useful for bone health. The best sources of dietary organic silicon are those mentioned above.

Boron

Is there a mineral that offers the same benefits as estrogen replacement therapy without side effects? Yes! In 1986 the consequence of major mineral metabolism in post-menopausal women was examined by the United States Department of Agriculture. It was found that boron supplementation markedly reduces the urinary excretion of calcium and magnesium.

Blood levels of estrogen in women taking boron rise to levels found in women on estrogen replacement therapy.

When we think of bone as the main storage site for boron as well as for calcium, the puzzle pieces begin to fit together.

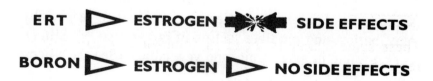

ERT ▷ ESTROGEN ⟶⟵ SIDE EFFECTS

BORON ▷ ESTROGEN ▷ NO SIDE EFFECTS

Boron is vital for the production of the active form of vitamin D and possibly for estrogen as well. The nutritionist who conducted the research for the United States Department of Agriculture, F. Nielson, PhD, believes that boron improves calcium retention. Additional studies confirm that boron enhances and mimics some effects of estrogen ingestion in postmenopausal women.[12]

Can we get enough boron from our foods? Not usually, according to three reasons offered by the *American Dietetic Association*: (1) excessive use of soluble chemical fertilizers; (2) levels of boron dropping in the last 50 years; (3) low concentrations affecting mineral metabolism.[13]

Alfalfa and kelp (also high in silicon) are excellent sources of boron. Under ideal growing conditions, spinach and snap beans contain significant quantities. Cabbage, lettuce, apples, leafy greens, legumes, and muskmelon leaves are next in line. But you would have to eat bagsful of these foods (for example, 5 apples or 14 pounds of lettuce) to get the necessary 3 milligrams of boron. The Food Tables on pages 255 to 261 list boron concentrations. Note the wide variation, dependent on soil and water conditions prevailing where and when the food in question was grown. (For more information on osteoporosis and bone health, see my booklet, *Startling New Facts About Osteoporosis*.)

A government study shows that people have fewer cavities in areas where water contains boron and other trace minerals.

These same elements found in abundance in cavity-free regions are sorely lacking in neighborhoods prone to a greater percentage of tooth decay.

Magnesium

Healthy bone is comprised of 20 percent calcium but only 0.1 percent magnesium. Small as that amount is, magnesium plays an important role in converting vitamin D to its active form. Magnesium is a powerful agent in the fixation of calcium.

> **High phosphorus levels in your diet can aggravate the symptoms of a magnesium deficiency.**

You can see how this business of nutrient dependency gets to be as fragile as a house of cards. Too much phosphorus affects magnesium, which affects vitamin D conversion, which affects calcium absorption, which affects bone health. And that's just one of many complex conditional pathways.

While the typical North American diet is deficient in magnesium, blood serum levels may appear to be normal due to self-regulating mechanisms that keep these levels up *at the expense of cellular magnesium.* So the best test for magnesium content is one that measures its level in your red blood cells.

> **Foods which have significant quantities of magnesium include eggs, liver, leafy greens, whole grains, legumes, seeds, almonds, black-eyed peas, curry, and mustard powder. How many of these foods have you eaten today?**

Stop for a moment and think about whether or not you have included high magnesium foods in your meals in the last few days. The leafy-green category does *not* include iceberg lettuce; the whole-grain category does *not* include cold, boxed cereals or white rice; and, obviously, curry and mustard powder would *not* be consumed in enough quantity to make a difference. Morning eggs (certified organic) and a handful of sprouted lentils usually help to assure my daily magnesium requirement. I supplement on other days.

Potassium

As already mentioned, the sodium-potassium pump that manages every cell in your body also impacts on premenstrual bloating. Part of the reason Asian women are comparatively free of our female afflictions may be their rich diets of dulse, kelp, and soybeans, which contain far more potassium than most other food substances. (For example, dulse, a seaweed, has 8,060 milligrams of potassium in 100 grams; a banana contains 370.)

Our processed-food diets disturb the natural ratios of sodium and potassium. In fact, it is virtually impossible to get enough potassium in our usual food supply to counter the sodium content of our foods—*even if we try*. That's why I recommend well-designed potassium supplementation. My preference is the liquid tonic preparations that have small amounts of various herbs and other whole-food-based nutrients, mixed with potassium.

Meanwhile, parsley, spinach, and asparagus are good foods of choice to add to your meals around "bloating time." My book, *Everything You Always Wanted to Know About Potassium But Were Too Tired to Ask,* answers many of the specific questions about potassium metabolism.

Chromium

Why do 98.5 percent of European people over the age of 50 have enough chromium, when only 25 percent of Americans in that same age group meet that standard? As for the rest of our population, short supplies of chromium subject almost every one of us to many problems, both subtle and serious. Too bad our American food supply has detached itself from nature.

Impaired glucose tolerance, high levels of circulating insulin, and insulin resistance are common dilemmas among contraceptive pill users and menopausal women.[14] Since chromium improves glucose tolerance and makes insulin more effective, this mineral is an excellent addition for the Pill user. (See Table 5 below.)

TABLE 5
SIGNS OF CHROMIUM DEFICIENCY

Chromium (200 micrograms daily) in the niacin-bound form, *chromium polynicotinate*, may be helpful if:

> ➤ You cannot lose weight
> ➤ You are under stress
> ➤ You overreact to ordinary circumstances
> ➤ You participate in athletics or aerobics
> ➤ You have any problems with blood-sugar metabolism (too high or too low)
> ➤ You sustain elevated cholesterol
> ➤ You are tired too often

Chromium supplements help to insure good health. Most of all, chromium polynicotinate can help to maximize energy potential.[15]

Zinc

Our appreciation for the significance of zinc becomes more pronounced with each research paper. All the carrots in the world would be useless for the many functions requiring vitamin A in the absence of sufficient zinc. Among other important attributes, zinc helps to transform beta-carotene into usable vitamin A, as stated above.

> **Perhaps it's not just an old wives' tale that oysters are especially good for libido. Oysters are a rich source of zinc!**

Consider Other Supplements

Hydrochloric Acid

Hydrochloric acid has already been cited as essential for bone/calcium metabolism. The least costly way to determine if you are deficient in hydrochloric acid is to purchase some in supplemental form at the health store. If you find after taking it that you can digest a food that formerly caused difficulty (pork chops, for example—if you still eat fatty meats), you can probably confirm your deficiency. A more accurate way is to consult your physician for scientific testing. You might point out to your physician that you are interested in your hydrochloric acid status because YOU KNOW that hydrochloric acid is necessary for good bone metabolism.

Gamma Linolenic Acid (GLA)

Essential fatty acids are just that—*essential*. They are important not only because they are a major component of the membranes surrounding all cells, but also because they help form *prostaglandins*, which are at the door of *every* cell, orchestrating many vital metabolic functions.[16]

One of the most powerful unsaturated fatty acids is *gamma linolenic acid* (GLA). GLA is found in very few foods and can only be manufactured in your body through a complex series of metabolic processes which decline in efficiency with age. In fact, most people have difficulty converting polyunsaturated oils to this activated form. Yet GLA is critical for the production of good-guy prostaglandins, which play a role in bone formation.

Fortunately, GLA is available in supplemental form. Sources of GLA are the oils of the seeds of black currants, borage, and primrose.

Are you recognizing a pattern here? Many of these nutrients seem to come from various fresh, natural foods. Eat with one nutrient in mind, and odds are you'll be supplying most of the others without any additional attention. It shouldn't come as any surprise that vegetarians (the *nutrient*-oriented type, not the *Twinkies* people) have higher bone density than age-matched meat eaters.

Other Supplements

This is far from a complete list of vitamins, minerals, and trace elements useful for avoiding the problems addressed here. Vitamin B_6 deficiency, for example, is critically important in the etiology of osteoporosis and may also play a key role in preventing arteriosclerosis and heart disease. In addition, B_6 gets good grades from those who suffer from PMS—perhaps because it helps to relieve depression and fluid retention. *And it also stimulates the production of progesterone!*

Under doctor's advisement, six grams of tryptophan were given daily to 13 women with severe PMS. Significant relief was experienced for depression, irritability, insomnia, and carbohydrate craving, with only mild side effects.

Then there's manganese, copper, and strontium (nonradioactive, of course!). But if your diet is heavily biased toward fresh and unprocessed foods and if you're paying attention to possible deficiencies that call for supplementation, it's unlikely that you'll miss *any* of the significant substances, not even those that are more obscure. A carefully selected quality multivitamin/mineral preparation plus a few supplements discussed on the following pages should help to cover all bases. *But please don't think of your supplements as a permanent replacement for a good diet!*

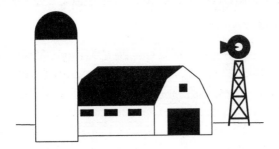

Whole foods are not mushed, mashed or mangled. They are the least harmful and the most nutritious.

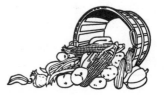

Select a Few Food-Type Supplements

I have always been a strong advocate of food-based supplements because these products run the gamut: *They contain nutrients already identified and those yet to be discovered.* They come in a natural matrix so that nutrients designed to "go together" are all present at roll call. Although by no means a complete list, garlic, acidophilus, flaxseed oil, beet crystals, kamut grass concentrate, and bee pollen are among those I like to recommend. I take several of these every day, varying my selection from time to time. Starting with garlic, the next few pages explain why.

EXTRA!!! The Times EXTRA!!!

GARLIC EXTRACT CURES CANCER IN TEST ANIMALS

Groups of hamsters were treated for up to fourteen weeks with a topical carcinogen. Prior to, during, and after treatment the test animals were also treated with a solution of an active ingredient found in garlic. The result? A significant reduction in tumor frequency, tumor burden, and lesion frequency.[17]

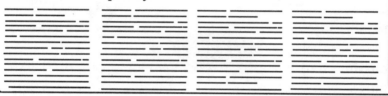

EXTRA!!! The Times EXTRA!!!

GARLIC PROTECTS AGAINST MAMMARY TUMORS

A study determined the influence of supplemental garlic powder on mammary tumors. Although food intake and weight gain were not influenced, the garlic powder significantly delayed the onset of tumors and reduced the total mammary tumor incidence. Consumption of garlic powder also significantly depressed the binding of carcinogens to mammary cell DNA.[18]

Garlic

Garlic has been used as a preventive and therapeutic agent for millennia (Sanskrit records document its use 5,000 years ago), perhaps because garlic's antimicrobial properties have been effective against a broad spectrum of bacteria, viruses, and fungi.

If you enjoy unusual stories about the use of special healing agents, note these about garlic: British soldiers applied garlic water directly to wounds during World War I; the Russians used garlic both internally and externally to speed healing during World War II.[19]

Deodorized forms of garlic may work almost as well as pure unadulterated fresh garlic. Probably the most important constituent of garlic is a chemical called *allicin*, the sulphurous and smelly substance that also seems to give garlic most of its outstanding medicinal qualities. Allicin is a natural antibiotic—it has even been compared favorably with penicillin for the treatment of certain classes of infections. But allicin in its active form is relatively scarce in fresh garlic. Its precursor, *alliin*, must be converted to allicin by the enzyme *allinase*. These two substances do not mix until the garlic is either digested or physically altered—explaining why the garlic smell becomes so strong when garlic is crushed.

One quality supplement comprised of garlic has gone through a long-term natural cold-aging process. The alliin is converted to beneficial sulfur compounds and the final product is odorless. The antimicrobial mechanisms of garlic supplements explain some of its beneficial effects. Research shows how garlic supplements increase natural immunity through its promotion of killer-cell activity. Test animals given this elixir are better able to resist the flu!

Flaxseed Oil

I like to tell the flaxseed oil story, so get ready for a little food history.

Once upon a time, every town and hamlet had its own oil mill. Many plants and seeds were used, but the favorite for producing oil was the flaxseed. It had a nutty, rich, almost creamy flavor, which (according to legend) tasted a lot like fresh butter.

As hamlets grew to towns and towns to cities, it became commonplace to have fresh oil delivered door-to-door, just as milk, eggs, and butter at a later time, or water today. Flaxseed oil was sold in small quantities and used only if fresh. The people understood just how its health-sustaining and therapeutic values worked best!

But oil-making practices changed with the use of machinery and specialization—efforts which made daily chores less arduous. Small presses were replaced with automated continuous-feed inventions. These were run at rates and pressures that raised the temperature of the oil far above the boiling point. Hydrocarbon solvents extracted more flax oil at a faster rate. The oil was also bleached, degummed, and deodorized to extend shelf life. Heat, light, air, and time provoked rancidity. So flaxseed oil, because it was no longer a "pure" and health-promoting product, eventually disappeared from the marketplace, taken over by corn and soy oil, among others.

As we gained knowledge, we became aware that fresh flaxseed oil contained two fatty acids not manufactured in the human body: *linoleic acid* (LA) and *linolenic acid* (LNA). The only way to get these fatty acids is to eat them. That's why they are called *essential*.

We also learned that LA and LNA are precursors—chemical building blocks of a large class of more elaborate fatty acids. These, in turn, are building blocks of literally thousands of enzymes, hormones, and prostaglandins—with many cellular functions, including bone formation. Arachidonic acid, made from LA, regulates viral infection and promotes resistance to toxins. Derivatives of LNA reduce the risk of fatal heart attacks and help to manufacture substances which control and limit blood platelet aggregation (sticking-together of blood platelets).

Flaxseed oil has a slow absorption rate. High in magnesium (necessary for vitamin D conversion), flax is also rich in lecithin, unmatched as a natural source of omega 3s, and has the components needed for good prostaglandin function.

Flax seed produces high concentrations of lignans, known to be protective against breast cancer and also to improve the ratios of progesterone and estradiol during menstruation.

An ample supply of LA and LNA is another way of insuring sufficient supplies of health-promoting nutrients—provided in abundance by fresh flaxseed oil. But what about this oil's rancidity problems? Shelf-life? Over-processing? All the detrimental effects of late twentieth century's current and careless foodways habits? Good news! It's BACK TO THE FUTURE: Today, you *can* get *pure, organic, unadulterated, non-rancid flaxseed oil* —in protective capsules—to add to your supplement regimen. (Be sure to refrigerate.) Or, you can buy an inexpensive small coffee grinder and whole flax seeds and grind as needed! (That's what I do.)

Red Beet Crystals

The rich, sweet, pungent red root of the beet is a wizard's brew of vitamins, minerals, and other important nutrients. I am especially fond of this supplement because it can disguise the taste of not-so-pleasant-tasting liquid nutrient blends.

Beets really are *good for your blood*— a statement assumed to be mythical, deriving from the blood-red color of its juice. Although our mothers and grandmothers couldn't possibly have known the scientific facts, there is something to the legend.

One of the problems with beets is that they require a lot of cooking. Vitamin B_6, so critical to most of the beneficial actions of the nutrients in beets, is sensitive to high temperatures. Since beets are usually boiled for anywhere from thirty minutes to two hours (at 212 degrees F), it's safe to say that a large portion of the original B_6 has departed as a result of the cooking process. Canned beets are subjected to even higher temperatures.

> **Crystallized beets, dissolved in water, capture the sweetness of beets and make potent nutrient mixtures delightfully palatable—without the losses incurred in the cooking process.**

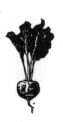 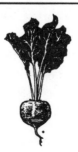 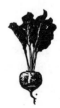

Pollen

Pollen is the male seed of flowers, and, like any seed, it contains across-the-board nutrients. Each pollen grain has from 1,000,000 to 5,000,000 pollen spores, all capable of reproducing the species.

This golden dust is comprised of thousands of enzymes and coenzymes—*many times more than in any other food.* An enzyme is a kind of catalyst, a substance that facilitates or promotes a chemical reaction, but is not itself consumed by the reaction. Enzymes can only be processed by a living organism.

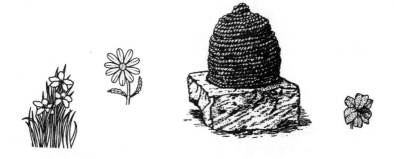

Dong Quai

Dr. Milner recommends *dong quai* (the herb *angelica*) because it is helpful for progesterone metabolism.[20] Dong quai serves as a pain and allergy reliever, with an effectiveness almost twice that of aspirin. (Dr. Milner also recommends folic acid to protect against deficiencies that may arise with the use of synthetic hormone therapy.)

Cautions:
➤ Dong quai should not be taken during pregnancy or for excessive menstrual flow.
➤ Vitamin E and folic acid in high doses should be regulated by your physician.

Kamut Sprouts

You are probably aware of the "green revolution" in food supplements. Young plants are powerful life forms containing high levels of nutrients, so the extracts of these shoots are gaining in popularity. Even more digestible than vegetables, young cereal grasses provide readily available vitamins, minerals, and enzymes.

The newest and most unique green food supplement available is *green kamut*. Green *what?* Kamut (pronounced ka-moot) is a grain whose history goes back to the cradle of civilization. According to folk lore, seeds recently discovered in an Egyptian pyramid germinated, bearing a bounty of nutrients. Although the story cannot be confirmed, the specialness of the product and one's imagination helps us to think there might be some truth in this tale.

A rich buttery flavor is among kamut's notable properties. An ancestor of our modern durum wheat, kamut is grown organically without having been subjected to the toxins and mutations of today's grains, and is less allergenic than other more familiar wheat products. Higher in protein, beta-carotene, and chlorophyll, kamut has been dubbed the new staff of life. For more information, see my newest book, *Kamut: An Ancient Food for a Healthy Future.*

Acidophilus

What? Add more bacteria to your gut? Yes, the good-guy variety, to crowd out bacteria of disreputable lineage. You can resist enemy invasion by entrenching your normal flora with healthful sentries. The easiest way to provide a settlement of proper bacteria is with acidophilus. A good acidophilus supplement loads a few billion acidophilus organisms per gram. The acidophilus bacteria "housekeep" in your intestines, creating an ecological system that helps to absorb nutrients and create new ones.

A similar helpful bacterium (*lactobacillus bulgaricus*, perhaps a second cousin once removed) is found in *viable* yogurt. Note the emphasis on viable; not all supermarket yogurts remain "live," and many have additives (emulsifiers, etc.) that are not in your best interest. Health store proprietors can direct you to the good brands.

Your great-grandmother probably produced another equally beneficial strain by "clabbering," or souring milk in her kitchen. Although not an American tradition, nearly every healthy society consumes a fermented or cultured food product of one type or another. Why? Because empirical observation shows that the addition of these foods is associated with disease prevention. At an international medical symposium, such products were noted as being important for the nutrition of people everywhere—especially in today's world. Fermentation is one of the most significant functions of the colonic flora.

There are more living entities in your flora than cells in your whole body. Acidophilus contributes favorably to this microflora, performing a wide variety of important functions in nutrition, immunology, and metabolism in general.

Long ago, the process was initiated by organisms present in raw foods, in the air, or on utensils. Today we use specific starter cultures and precise conditions of time and temperature, insuring superior products and microbial safety.

Chinese Medicine

Herbal medicines can also be useful to help you journey through menopause. With a little knowledge, you can make educated choices about using herbs to improve health as well as to reduce common menopausal symptoms. See the section starting on page 233 for an account of helpful Chinese herbal medicine described by Dr. Herb Kandel.

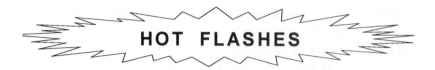

HOT FLASHES

➤ Flax seed enhances progesterone/estradiol ratios during menstruation.
Clinical Endocrinology Metabolism, 1993[21]

➤ Multivitamin and mineral supplements containing a broad range of vitamins (A, B_2, B_5, B_6, B_9, E) and minerals (Cr, Cu, Mg, Se, Si, Zn) appear to be justified for menopausal women.
Francaise de Gynecologie et D Obstetrique, 1990[22]

➤ Complete multi's work better for protecting bone marrow cells which have been exposed to carcinogenic and genetic hazards than vitamin C alone.
Mutation Research, 1992[23]

➤ Vitamin C is required for connective tissues such as cartilage and bone.
Nutrition Reviews, 1992[24]

➤ Vitamin C decreases the frequency of the pesticide-induced changes in bone marrow.
Mutation Research, 1993[25]

➤ Vitamin C increases collagen synthesis, and thus, inhibits cancer cell metabolism and proliferation.
Experimental and Toxicologic Pathology, 1992[26]

➤ Toxins which would normally cause bone cells to fragment are protected by vitamin C.
Food and Chemical Toxicology, 1992[27]

➤ Magnesium deficiency plays a role in the etiology of premenstrual syndrome.
Acta Obstetricia et Gynecology Scandinavica, 1994[28]

➤ Vitamin C improves bone deformities associated with displaced fractures.
Laboratory Animal Care, 1992[29]

➤ Calcium absorption may be impaired by decreased ability of kidneys to produce hormonal vitamin D.
Annual Review of Nutrition, 1990[30]

➤ Decreased bone mineral content is prevalent in infants whose mothers were calcium- and magnesium-deficient during pregnancy.

American College of Nutrition, 1992[31]

➤ Calcium excretion is nutrition-dependent and is influenced by vitamin D status.

Minerva Medica, 1992[32]

➤ Vitamin D influences bone density.

British Medical Jnl, 1992[33]

➤ The active vitamin D component is essential for calcium absorption and bone health.

Jnl of Internal Medicine, 1992[34]

➤ Boron is relatively nontoxic.

Archives of Environmental Contamination and Toxicology, 1990[35]

➤ One sign of boron deprivation is depressed bone magnesium.

Biological Trace Element Research, 1988[36]✝

➤ Boron is important for optimal calcium and, thus, bone metabolism.

Biological Trace Element Research, 1990[37]✝

➤ Dietary lack of boron and silicon may result in suboptimal function and composition of both bone and brain.

Asociacion Medica de Puerto Rico, 1991[38]

➤ Boron deficiency may cause arthritis.

Nutrition and Health, 1991[39]

➤ Magnesium depletion leads to calcium deficiency in the blood.

Magnesium Research, 1992[40]

➤ Magnesium plays a major role in bone formation.

American Jnl of Clinical Nutrition, 1964[41]

➤ Silicon is essential for the metabolism of connective and bone tissue.

Clinical Therapeutics, 1991[42]

➤ Silicon is a major constituent of the cells concerned with bone growth.

Science of the Total Environment, 1988[43]

➤ Daily administration of vitamin D_3 significantly reduces the incidence of nonvertebral fractures.

Revue du Rhumatisme, 1994[44]

UPDATES

Calcif Tissue International 1997 Jan;60(1):115-8
Treatment with active vitamin D metabolites is very effective in slowing fast trabecular bone loss in osteoporotic and osteopenic patients.

American Jnl of Clinical Nutrition 1997 Mar;65(3):803-13
Dietary boron affects mineral metabolism, especially in those subjected to nutritional stressors. There is no evidence of toxic boron accumulation over time.

Fundamental Applied Toxicol 1997 Feb;35(2):205-15
Boron consumption increases compression resistance at exposure levels substantially below those that were previously reported to be reproductively toxic.

Osteoporosis International 1996,6(6):453-61
The increase in bone density in response to magnesium therapy in gluten sensitive people suggests that magnesium depletion may be one factor contributing to osteoporosis in any one suffering from gluten sensitivity.

Jnl Pediatr Gastroterol Nutr 1996 Jul;23(1):8-12
Over a range of usual calcium intakes, during the rapid-bone-growth period in childhood and early adolescence, urinary calcium appears relatively unaffected by calcium intake and is most strongly associated with urinary sodium levels. [A good reason to keep those salted chips away from your children!]

Journal of Nutrition 1996 Apr; 126(4 Suppl):1159S-64S
Aging, sunscreen use and the change in the zenith angle of the sun can dramatically affect your production of vitamin D3. Vitamin D insufficiency is now being recognized as a major cause of bone disease.

Jnl of Clinical Endocrinol Metab 1996 Jun;81(6):2017-20
The peak time for bone calcium deposition is in the premenarcheal and perimenarcheal time period.

~~ ENDNOTES ~~ *The fantasy continues...*

Throughout these pages, I have used the words *complicated* and *complex* time and again. As our fantasy continues, we can see why: The interrelationships of metabolic processes are more than overwhelming—one nutrient dependent on another, conditional to another, subservient to yet another; one *hormone* influencing another, and so on.

Now we see how our thyroid and steroid hormones are related. Much more than kissing cousins, they are part of a multitiered puppet show. The pituitary pulls the thyroid strings while the thyroid, a pinkish "bow tie" sitting on our windpipe, manipulates the bone-growth strings. We watch, as our thyroid dances to the pituitary's tune, producing hormones to deposit or reduce calcium in our bones or in our blood.

Now the act changes. We see the master puppeteer, the hypothalamus, maneuvering the pituitary. We watch as a surge of events crashes through our body—*the immediate physical reactions to stress.*

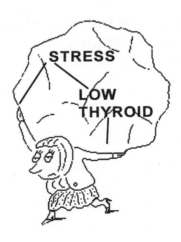

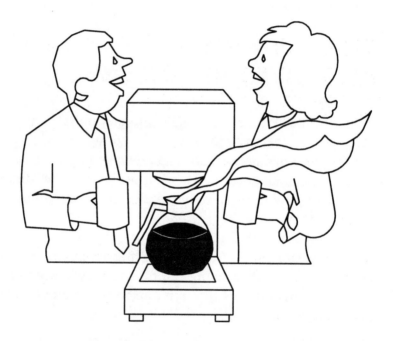

We emptied the fridge of all the junk food last night. Now there's nothing left but the light bulb.

13

THE THYROID
AND STRESS CONNECTIONS

THE SYNERGY OF ALL BODY PARTS

THE THYROID CONNECTION

The head bone *is* connected to the neck bone—a concept clearly demonstrated by the association between thyroid function and seemingly separate metabolic actions. It's no news that there is a direct correlation between immune responses and thyroid function. But important ties also exist between thyroid function and sex hormones,[1] between thyroid hormone and progesterone receptor levels,[2] and between thyroid performance and bone metabolism.[3] And that's just the beginning.

Low thyroid hormone translates to poor progesterone management, which means disturbed menstrual and menopausal control! Low thyroid hormone, for example, invariably means low progesterone levels in the luteal phase.

Thyroid hormone interacts with FSH (the follicle-stimulating hormone). So adequate circulating levels of thyroid hormone is one factor responsible for successful induction of ovulation.[4] The growth of the mammary gland is also regulated by a complex interaction of thyroid and steroid hormones.[5]

> The frequent occurrence of spontaneous abortion in early pregnancy may be caused by inadequate thyroid hormone.[6]

How do you know if low thyroid function is your problem? Not easily. Frustration about the nonspecific clinical manifestations of a low thyroid output and confusion about the many tests to check for this disorder are commonplace.[7] Signs and symptoms of thyroid deficiency and interpretation of thyroid tests become even more difficult as we get older. As we age, we are more likely to develop problems with fluid and electrolyte balances (more of what we *don't* need at menopause!), which are tied to thyroid function. A decreased sensitivity of the thirst mechanism may be an important contributor to these imbalances.[8]

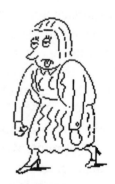

Fatigue may be an indication of a low-functioning thyroid. For symptom-free menstruation and menopausal integrity, thyroid function must be optimal.

One good indication of low thyroid outlay is *cold intolerance*—cold hands and feet. Other benchmarks are tendencies to weight gain, dry skin, brittle nails, chronic fatigue, and even constipation.

The best telltale, however, is to check your pituitary hormone levels rather than your thyroid secretions. Here's why:

Thyroid-stimulating hormone (TSH) is secreted by your pituitary. Very simply, if you require more thyroid hormone, your brain signals your pituitary, which then signals your thyroid to produce more thyroid hormone. High TSH translates to your pituitary giving your thyroid the message to produce *more* thyroid hormone. Low TSH is an indication that your thyroid is attempting to close down; it's overproducing.

But the problem is that you may have low TSH as the result of taking an excess of thyroid hormone, prescribed because you had a low thyroid hormone output to begin with! According to researchers reporting in *Postgraduate Medicine*, the TSH assay is the single most important test in the diagnosis and treatment of hypothyroidism (low thyroid production).[9]

Because proper thyroid function has such a profound effect on so many organ systems, physicians often prescribe medication for those who don't produce enough thyroid hormone on their own. But treatment, if not watched carefully, can be a double-edged sword.

> Too much thyroid hormone increases bone turnover, which, in turn, may lead to bone loss from your spine and hip.[10]

Studies have shown that treatment of a low thyroid condition results in loss of cortical and trabecular bone, placing you at risk for osteoporosis.[11,12] The effect of thyroid therapy on bone mineral density has prompted recommendations to prescribe doses of thyroxine at lower levels.[13] If you are on thyroid hormone therapy, discuss this potential problem—its advantages and disadvantages—with your physician.

MEMOS

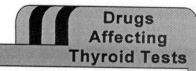

Drugs
Affecting
Thyroid Tests

Drugs Affecting Results of Tests to Determine Thyroid Function

Corticosteroids
suppress TSH; block conversion of thyroid hormones (T_4 to T_3)

Cough medications
can induce hypothyroidism if preparation contains iodine

Estrogens
falsely increase total T_4 level

Dilantin
decreases total T_4 level

Salicylates (aspirin)
decrease T_4 level

You can see how drugs may affect thyroid test results, thereby contributing to misleading conclusions.

R_x

MEMOS

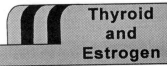

Thyroid and Estrogen

Thyroid Function and Estrogen Activity

One of your thyroid hormones helps to regulate estrogen. If you are hypothyroid and not secreting enough of this hormone, you increase the risk of having higher circulating estrogen throughout your body.

With a sleepy thyroid, there is a dramatic shift from high to low estrogen at the time of menopause. This extreme shift is apparent in many women who develop osteoporosis. They have trouble making estrogen themselves because of the previously high circulating levels.

Adequate (but not excessive) levels of iodine, zinc, and copper are necessary for the conversion of thyroid hormones.

THE STRESS CONNECTION

I suppose I've always been interested in the relation of mind and body, growing up as I did in a culture that separated them distinctly...Every day in this divided world of mind and body, our language betrayed the limitations of our categories. Widow Brown must have died of a broken heart—she never got sick until after her husband was gone.

So begins the odyssey of Bill Moyers, a respected journalist, as he confirms that mind and body are connected—something the sages have known for centuries. As suggested by the opening statement in his book, *Healing and the Mind*, the concept that thoughts and feelings influence health has often gone by the wayside in our world of specialization.

We are, however, coming closer to understanding some of the "magic" responsible for the mind/body fusion. This connection may be referred to as grandma's insight, but the professionals call it *psychoneuroimmunology*—a coming together of psychology, neurology, and immunology—a kind of therapy that is not old-fashioned but is undeniably old.

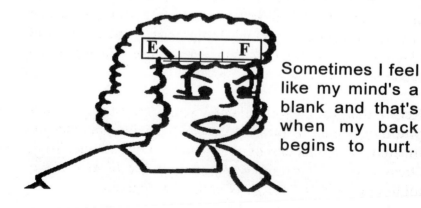

Sometimes I feel like my mind's a blank and that's when my back begins to hurt.

Advances in contemporary medicine have allowed an exploration of the human mind in ways never thought possible before. As explained in *Lancet*:

> *Many of the functions of the mind, such as perception, learning, speech, memory, sleep, dreams, mood regulation, and pain control are now being understood in terms of physiological and/or biochemical phenomena. Control by the brain over other body functions is known to occur through various processes.*
>
> *Immune cells can secrete substances which in the brain are known to alter sleep, appetite, and hormone secretion.*[14]

Levels of many hormones increase as compensatory reactions. Additional cortisol secretion helps to stabilize blood sugar levels—as occurred, for example, following the Chernobyl accident in response to the radiation exposure. This is just one way our body uses hormones in an attempt to help us adapt to unusual situations.[15]

Can you actually alter hormone metabolism because of how you *think* or how you *feel*? This is a distinct possibility as long as your brain and other body systems continue talking to each other. Don't brain/body interactions take place when you respond with tears while viewing a sad scene in a movie?

Recall that your hypothalamus sends messages to your pituitary, which in turn influences your adrenals and ultimately the production of estrogen and progesterone. Well, stress begins its destructive action at the level of your midbrain—and the target is your hypothalamus.

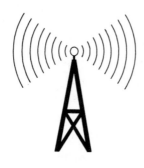

Your hypothalamus works like the dispatching station of a telecommunications center. Once it receives notice of an uncomfortable situation it sends stimulating impulses to its entire territory. This gland is theorized to be the primary trigger of aging, disease, and health for the whole organism.

We also know that stress affects fatty acid metabolism, which affects cholesterol, which affects progesterone, which affects cortisol, which affects YOU. This hormonal relay system may be the reason why women report feeling so much better emotionally when they start using natural progesterone, and why arthritis symptoms disappear.

When your adrenals are overworked (from either emotional or physical stress) and can't produce enough of the stress-relieving hormones, your body converts existing progesterone to these hormones. Zap! There goes your progesterone.

If you feel stressed because your mother-in-law tries to tell you what to do, or your daughter-in-law won't listen to your words of wisdom, or your teenager is causing you grief because he or she is "adolescing," your calcium may diminish in relation to hormone levels.[16]

So we can explain a few facts about how stress relates to PMS and menopausal symptoms. It's not just mind over matter; it's mind *controlling* matter: how you feel can change the natural direction of metabolic processes and alter biological patterns that are clearly identifiable.

It has been shown that the combination of stress and junk foods causes women to miss their periods. Take them off the junk food and the periods come back, even in the presence of the same stress![17] This is in accordance with my belief that *when your stress mechanisms are well nourished they do not break down!* If stress is less destructive under given circumstances, let's work with those particulars, i.e., *better diet.*

Easier said than done! Diet and lifestyle changes are difficult. At the very least, consider the alternative of taking supplements and adding natural progesterone—especially at times of *super* stress.

Keep in mind the associations between:
> ➢ **Destructive stress and junk food**
> ➢ Destructive stress and lack of nutrients
> ➢ Destructive stress and natural progesterone deficiencies

Learning simple stress-relieving mechanisms to help block hurtful events can also help. Books and tapes describing such exercises are widely available. You probably have ample opportunity to practice these techniques when you are late and find yourself stuck in a major traffic jam.

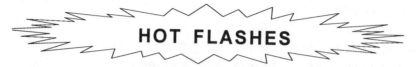

HOT FLASHES

➤ A strong thyroid-adrenal interdependence has been demonstrated time and again.
Febs Letters, 1991[18]

➤ Adrenal substances respond to emotional strain.
Jnl of Neurochemistry, 1992[19]

➤ Stress causes abnormal enlargement of the adrenals and a detrimental change in the thymus.
Neuroscience and Behavioral Physiology, 1992[20]

➤ Emotional stress results in reactions in the hypothalamus and adrenals, among other problems.
Kardiologiia, 1992[21]

➤ Estrogens may be released from the adrenals and/or ovaries during psychological stress, contributing to excesses.
Neuroscience and Biobehavioral Reviews, 1992[22]

UPDATES

Thyroid 1996 Apr;6(2):75-8
Overzealous thyroxine replacement which produces subclinical hyperthyroidism may result in an increase in bone turnover.

New England Journal of Medicine 1996;335:1176-1181
Depression may increase a woman's risk for brittle or broken bones. Bone density was 10 to 14 percent lower in depressed women. [Estrogen contributes to depression.]

1996 *American College of Obstetricians and Gynecologists*
Seventy percent of new mothers experience mood swings of some form (crying spells, sleeplessness, loss of appetite, irritability, anger or an inability to make decisions). If the depression lasts longer than two weeks, it is most likely hormonally induced.

~~ ENDNOTES ~~ *The fantasy continues...*

The next segment of my fantasy doesn't require any yet-to-be-discovered technology. It does, however, require an extraordinary imagination. Picture, if you will, all the women for whom synthetic estrogens and progestins have been prescribed. They descend, en masse, on their doctors' doorsteps, demanding that their prescriptions be rewritten for *natural* progesterone. And—remember, this is fantasy—the doctors happily cooperate and rewrite all the prescriptions, even though the application of natural progesterone cream is so safe, no prescription is necessary!

The crowds on the physicians' doorsteps and in their waiting rooms increase as the good news about the use of natural progesterone for conditions other than PMS, menopausal symptoms, and osteoporosis becomes more widespread. Most of the ten million women now on these synthetic risk-laden drugs shift gears.

Or the assemblage decreases as women learn about self-help. Even better, they may dwindle because they have learned about prevention.

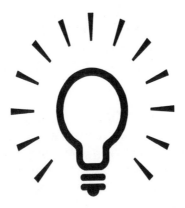

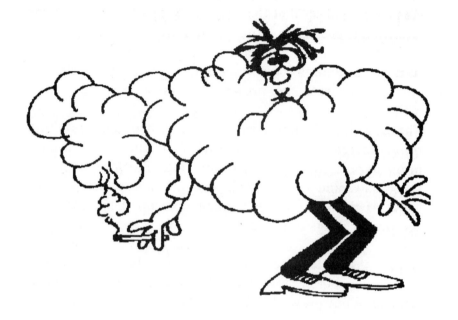

Why do you think I got that letter from
the EPA warning me about my contribution to indoor pollution?

14

PROGESTERONE TREATMENT

PROGESTERONE FOR BALANCE

If you were to tell me that you've done all the good things listed in the food and supplement chapters most of your life, I'd be very surprised if you had a problem with PMS, menopause, or osteoporosis. I'd also be very surprised if you were telling the truth! Let's be realistic—almost nobody in this society can follow such a strict regimen of prohibitions. Most of us need help! And that help may come in the form of a plant-based progesterone-like substance plus synergistic herbs.

The word progesterone was first proposed by William Allen and George Corner in 1934, when they isolated this newly discovered sex hormone. Since then, more than 5,000 plants have been identified as containing substances with progesterone-like chemistry. In 1943, Russel Marker successfully manufactured progesterone from the Mexican yams. With minor conversion in the laboratory, *diosgenin*, the Mexican yam extract, has been made to match natural progesterone exactly. But the manufacture of cortisone and progestogins from the same raw materials attracted far more attention. The neglect of progesterone led Dr. Dalton to refer to it as "the forgotten hormone."[1]

MEMOS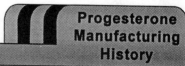

History of the Manufacture of Progesterone
(Outside the Human Body)

The principal source of the steroid chemical nucleus used in the drug industry is the plant kingdom. In the not too distant past, however, the source was the gonads and adrenal glands of animals that were used as food by people. Because the amount of hormone present in these glands was extremely small, large quantities of glands were required to isolate very minute amounts. For example, one laboratory extracted 625 kilograms of ovaries from 50,000 sows in order to obtain 20 milligrams of pure crystalline progesterone.

Today, the steroid industry represents the culmination of the efforts of many scientists. Plant species rich in steroidal substances have been discovered. Included is the Mexican yam. Using these *sapogenins*, the cost scaled down considerably. A vast amount of research resulted in improvement of the basic procedures over the years.

In addition to Mexican yams, diosgenin is also derived from soybean products (recall the lack of PMS and menopausal symptoms among Asians), and, occasionally from animal sources. In France, it is taken from human placenta.

The success of many practitioners has helped us to catch up with this hormone. The spotlight has been turned back in progesterone's direction.

When is the use of progesterone appropriate? *Like nearly all of us*, you may be among the women who could benefit from assistance. Reports of improved well-being with the use of transdermal natural progesterone are impressive. Less anxiety and depression, increased vitality and reduced sleep disturbances—not to mention enhanced libido—are all benefits of a product with a track record of total safety![2] Add to this a handful of herbs used for centuries to balance women's hormones, and the effects of the progesterone become even more enhanced and more far-reaching—including the elimination of migraines, relief of arthritic pain, return of joint flexibility, breaking up of fatty tumors, and the disappearance of cysts and fibroids.

Are you already on estrogen replacement therapy? Do you want to bail out? A slow weaning process is recommended, preferably under a physician's care. If you are on Premarin, for example, you may be advised to cut down your intake by 10 to 15 percent each month simply by skipping days. (Skipping days may work better than dividing the tablets only because they are difficult to split.) As for patches, they can be worn for shorter periods of time, gradually diminishing the duration of their application. Injections can be spaced further apart, and eventually phased out.

If, however, you have made the decision to continue or to begin the traditional form of hormone or estrogen replacement therapy (HRT or ERT), it should be clear that natural progesterone used in conjunction with estrogen could be beneficial. Most physicians now prescribe oral progestin with the oral estrogen pill. Try to avoid synthetic progestin—*ask your physician to recommend natural progesterone.*

Most nutrition-aware physicians prescribe estrogen for meno-pausal patients only if other treatments fail to reduce symptoms. A rare occurrence, they recommend just enough estrogen to cut problems to a tolerable degree—not necessarily to eliminate them; they want to keep the dose low. But they agree that natural progesterone is an absolute MUST to accompany estrogen therapy. Dr. Robert Atkins of New York City also recommends high doses of folic acid plus boron for anyone on estrogen replacement therapy.[3] (Again: high doses of folic acid should be taken only under doctor's advisement.)

Another problem with synthetic progestins involves glucose (blood sugar) metabolism. You may experience a drop in blood sugar if your progesterone is low. Low blood sugar causes the sensation of hunger, and you know how that feels—you're ready to jump on your child or spouse for no reason. This scenario occurs with the use of synthetic progestins because the synthetics do *not* convert to cor-ticosteroids. Natural progesterone, on the other hand, is converted into corticosteroid hormones by your adrenal glands, thus avoiding the problem by helping to regulate your blood sugar metabolism.

To add insult to injury, synthetic progestins lower your production of natural progest-erone levels.

Neils H. Lauersen, M.D., of New York's Mt. Sinai Medical Center, advises that synthetic progestins may inhibit the concentration of natural progesterone, so hormone imbal-ances—which may be "off" to begin with—are worsened with their use.[4]

> Any standard medical text explains that estrogen's maximum benefit for osteoporosis is no more than a temporary reduction in the rate of osteoporotic bone resorption.

Physicians are influenced, albeit inadvertently, by drug-company advertising rather than by information in their own textbooks. When you understand the functions of the osteoblasts and osteoclasts (as explained earlier), you can talk about bone loss to your physician with more knowledge. You might even tell your doctor that you know that natural progesterone stimulates osteoblasts, and that synthetic estrogen restrains osteoclasts, but only slightly, and only temporarily. Yes, you understand these functions now.

Chances are you now know as much about natural progesterone metabolism as most physicians. Don't hesitate to show these chapters to your doctor, pointing out the extensive medical journal citations and clinical validations included throughout and at the back of this book.

When you intervene with synthetic estrogen you're adding a powerful hormone that has a direct effect on tissue all over your body. But progesterone is more of an intermediate building block. You're giving your endocrine system a tool to work with—leaving your natural control and regulation mechanisms in place. That explains why it's so much safer to use natural progesterone than estrogen. Remember our discussion of the huge dose of progesterone you made for yourself during pregnancy? Far from being harmful, it helped you feel great, even euphoric. In addition, studies show that natural progesterone helps to prevent or reverse osteoporosis whether or not supplemental estrogen is used.[5,6]

Recall that one traditional problem with the use of natural progesterone in the oral form is that your liver attempts to protect you from dietary hormones with first-pass removal. Dr. Dalton lamented the lack of an easy way of getting progestins into the bloodstream. She wrote:

> *For many doctors progesterone is a forgotten hormone so far as treatment is concerned, and many doctors who use estrogen and know its possibilities and limitations are shy of using progesterone. Progesterone cannot be taken by mouth, as it is too quickly broken down in the liver, so it has to be given in other ways such as pessaries (tablets to be inserted into the vagina), suppositories (for use in the anus), injections, or implants. Recent work in India suggested that it is absorbed into the bloodstream when given by nasal administration. So who knows, we may yet be using it in aerosols or nasal sprays.*[7]

There is a way to circumvent the difficulty! Wild yam extract and natural progesterone are formulated in a cream base that may also contain aloe vera, vitamin E, jojoba and/ or avocado oils, burdock root extract, Siberian ginseng, chamomile, and/or even black cohosh extract—plus cream protectors. Spreading the cream over an area of skin is the method of application, so that the hormone can enter your blood *transdermally* (through your skin). The cream leaves no trace after a few minutes. Some oil-based liquids also appear to sidestep the problem.

In *Cancer Causes and Control*, researchers advise that women currently using unopposed estrogen, estrogen and synthetic progestins, or synthetic progestins alone, are all at increased risk for breast cancer compared with never-users, and that the addition of synthetic oral progesterone (more accurately, *progestin*) does *not* remove the increased risk observed with current use of unopposed estrogen.[8] This is typical of an error in the use of the word *progesterone*, an inaccuracy made by many physicians. It cannot be overemphasized that side effects stem from *synthetic* progestins, not from *natural* progesterone. Again, the word progesterone refers to the specific molecule made by your ovary and adrenals, and not to the numerous synthetic substitutes.

As Dr. Lee explains:

> *There are no known side effects from natural progesterone which, as should be obvious to all, is the preferred form to use if supplementation is to be given.*
>
> *Estrogen increases the risk of breast cancer over time and this risk can be reduced by progesterone, but not by all progestins. Both estrogen and most progestins increase intracellular sodium and water, leading to hypertension, whereas progesterone acts to prevent intracellular sodium and water, thus preventing hypertension and sparing the heart. Some progestins increase blood lipids, but natural progesterone does not. [Many physicians and researchers] confuse the synthetic progestins with natural progesterone.[9]*

Is it any wonder that breast cancer has increased so rapidly in recent years? Victims in the United States alone could fill a 747 every day. And on every third day, the equivalent of a 747 full of women die from this avoidable disease.

Should you self-treat with natural progesterone? Until recently, the short answer to this question was "No." Safe creams now provide viable options.

Is it okay to use progesterone creams without medical supervision? Although it's always best to have the guidance of a nutrition-oriented MD, clinical experience suggests an affirmative answer. Daily application to soft-skin areas (breasts, neck, face, stomach, inside area of thighs, and upper inner arms) are recognized as safe. Mexican yam extract with a small amount of progesterone, plus synergistic herbal extracts (discussed previously), mixed in a cream base, appears to be both risk free and very effective.

Using a different part of your body each of four nights, and then repeating the areas of application, may provide more efficient delivery. Once fat cells are saturated with progesterone, they may not accept any more (especially if you are using high-dose formulas). If you can't recall your last contact site, not to worry! Finger tips are sensitive—the minute you apply the cream to your finger, the absorption process commences.

If you are concerned about any infertility effect, apply the cream from Day 15 to Day 25 of your cycle. However, using the low-dose progesterone creams with the herbal additions appears to eliminate the chances of progesterone-caused infertility.

Some women experience immediate relief; others find that it may take from one to four months to turn things around. Remember, this is a natural product, not a drug.

Just as we recommend starting any new supplement in small amounts, we suggest starting the cream in small quantities, too, especially if you are going to apply it to your face.

PROGESTERONE FOR MENOPAUSE

When using preparations that follow FDA recommendations (a maximum of 10 milligrams of natural progesterone per two-ounce jar), it's not entirely necessary to stop application at any time. (This assumes that your low-dose product also contains synergistic herbs.) Many women just don't feel as good on days during which they stop application. Your body is not only responding to the progesterone, but also to the phytoprogesterones, the phytoestrogens, and other miscellaneous benefits of the additional herbs.

If, however, you are using a high-dose preparation and want to treat menopausal symptoms, and you are still menstruating, ¼ teaspoon twice a day is appropriate from Day 7 to Day 20 (during which time ovulation should occur, usually on Day 14); then use ½ teaspoon twice a day from Day 21 to the start of your period. If you are no longer menstruating, don't apply cream the first week of the month (Days 1 through 6), and then proceed as above.

For hot-flash or night-sweat crises, apply ¼ to ½ teaspoon at 15-minute intervals for one hour or until flashes disappear. A severe case? Apply more! A jar's worth of the low-dose progesterone variety will not give you as much "hormone" as a single dose of risk-laden synthetic progestins. Recall that most herbs work *adaptogenically*, and generally do not continue their action when no longer required.

Even though you may never have experienced menopausal symptoms (the result of a prudent lifestyle), you may still be subject to stresses and to xenoestrogen exposure. We are using 3½-million-year-old genes in a late twentieth century world. I know I cannot get enough natural progesterone or its precursors even if I continue to eat the best food available without help—regardless of my heroic efforts.

PROGESTERONE FOR VAGINAL DRYNESS

For vaginal dryness, ¼ to ½ teaspoon of cream applied intravaginally once a day helps immeasurably. Also insert a vitamin E capsule, 400 IU, intravaginally, once a day. (No need to break open the capsule; the pH of your body will do the job.) With this treatment, women report the problem remedied within a very short time.

PROGESTERONE FOR OSTEOPOROSIS

For mild osteoporosis, apply ¼ teaspoon twice a day. Severe osteoporosis or broken bones in the past? 2 ounces or more a month.

When asked how long a woman should use the cream, Dr. Lee says, "Until you are 96. Then we'll see."

PROGESTERONE FOR STRESS

A vivacious, sparkly woman came up to me at a meeting and said, "I never knew there was anything wrong with me until I started using the cream." My own niece had recently been assigned a high-powered political position. Her therapist suggested Prozac to help her get through her inability to cope with the new pressures. After three weeks of cream application, Carol called to say, "Aunt Betty, I never knew it was possible to feel this good."

In a more extreme case, a woman confessed that she had actually investigated three ways of committing suicide. Now she relates her plight with both tears and laughter—the result of her renewed prespective on life, thanks to progesterone cream.

Recall that progesterone is responsible for the manufacture of cortisol and other adrenal gland hormones.

PROGESTERONE FOR PMS

The damage done by half a lifetime of environmental assaults (not to mention your mother's lifestyle before and during *her* pregnancy) may be insurmountable if you use only the sometimes-blunt and slow-acting tools of lifestyle change. Besides, following the perfect diet and exercise routine may be impossible for good reasons. Don't feel guilty. Feel better! Natural progesterone could make the difference.

Varying degrees of PMS have been treated successfully with the use of natural progesterone cream by many physicians. Esther Kirk, MD, in Westwood Village, California, notes that several PMS patients refer to progesterone cream as their "miracle cream."[10] Psychiatrist Louis Marx reports, "I have not encountered any substance which is more effective than progesterone in relieving PMS."[11] Dr. Serafina Corsello says, "This treatment has made a tremendous difference. I personally wouldn't be without my progesterone cream." Dr. Richard Kunin says that some of his patients experience PMS relief in less than 15 minutes.[12] Dr. Lee says, "The beneficial change in the quality of life with progesterone cream is remarkable."[13] Martin Milner, ND, of Portland, Oregon, is astounded by physicians who prescribe estrogen with apparent abandon—when it's progesterone that is more frequently deficient in pre-, peri-, and postmenopausal women.

The practitioners listed above were pioneers. In the last few years, hundreds of other physicians have joined the bandwagon. I recently sent a questionnaire to a group of nutrition-oriented MDs, and more than 75 percent responded, confirming that they did indeed use progesterone cream with herbs as a major part of their treatment for women of all ages, and for all hormone-related complaints.

General instructions for PMS: For low-dose-progesterone-herbal formulas, applying ¼ to ½ teaspoon daily usually works, but your own judgment with experimentation is the best gauge. At a recent symposium, attended by physicians who have been observing patients who use progesterone cream, the concensus was that *how you feel* is the best benchmark for use. (Never mind those blood and saliva tests.)

For the more potent formulas, no cream should be applied from Day 1 (start of period) to Day 14; apply 1/8 teaspoon twice a day from Day 14 to Day 17; apply ¼ teaspoon twice a day from Day 18 to Day 22; apply ½ teaspoon twice a day on Day 23 to the day your period starts.

For cramping at the onset of a period, apply ½ teaspoon of cream to your abdomen every 30 minutes until cramping subsides. For PMS migraines, the doctors suggest ¼ to ½ teaspoon of the cream applied to the back of your neck and across your forehead and temples. Larger doses of natural progesterone are recommended if needed to counter the PMS culprit—namely, *high amounts of estrogen.*

How does natural progesterone work to relieve the burdensome symptoms of PMS? Turn back to Figure 6 on page 50, which shows the relative levels of estrogen and progesterone during a normal 28-day cycle, with Day 1 defined as the first day of menstruation. Notice the progesterone build-up after ovulation (normally at Day 14), which tapers off again before Day 1 of the next cycle. PMS generally occurs between ovulation and the beginning of menstruation, when serum levels of progesterone should be highest (days 14 to 28 on the chart).

The average progesterone level after ovulation is lower in PMS sufferers than in those without symptoms.

We don't know exactly why progesterone deficiency occurs. Your ovaries may not be producing enough. Perhaps you're deficient in one of the ovary-controlling hormones of the hypothalamus or pituitary gland. *Or it may be a problem of too much estrogen compared with a normal amount of progesterone*—in which case the addition of natural progesterone helps to normalize the ratio.

Progesterone deficiency may be a simple reaction to stress. Without progesterone to thicken uterine walls in preparation for a fertilized egg, pregnancy is unlikely. It makes sense— would you really want to get pregnant during a time of high stress? I find this explanation attractively uncomplicated, but we don't really know if it's totally correct.

What we *do* know is that there is evidence that natural progesterone supplementation works to alleviate PMS in the majority of cases. We also know that synthetic progestins, because they inhibit the concentration of natural progesterone, heighten the imbalance of hormones and intensify PMS symptoms. A few of the progestins in the marketplace are actually 2,000 times more potent than natural progesterone, which may be why some of these drug preparations can make you feel worse than others.

Progesterone treatments have been accepted so completely in Great Britain that, in three different murder trials, women have been "sentenced" to take progesterone. The defense? They committed violent crimes because they were premenstrual. Instead of going to jail, these women were remanded to their pharmacists.[14]

Application tip: Apply a hot cloth to the site of application before applying the cream. This opens pores for better absorption. Vaginal application also enhances absorption.

PROGESTERONE AND OTHER APPLICATIONS

Sex steroids affect the anatomy and physiology of many organ systems. Following are examples of the benefits of progesterone, apart from those demonstrated for PMS and menopause.

Pregnancy

What about progesterone supplementation during pregnancy? There's intriguing data about increased intelligence that sounds almost too exciting to be true. An abstract of a paper that appeared in the *British Journal of Psychiatry* follows:

> *Children whose mothers received prenatal progesterone have been shown to be advanced in development at one year and to have greater academic achievement at nine to ten years. This study compares the educational attainments at 17 to 20 years of 34 progesterone children with 37 normal and 12 toxemic controls. More progesterone children continued schooling after 16 years compared with controls; higher proportion left school with..."A" level passes; the average number of passes per child was greater; and more obtained a university place. The best academic results were in those whose mothers had received over five grams of prenatal progesterone and for whom administration commenced before the sixteenth week and for whom treatment lasted longer than eight weeks.*

Objective measures of intelligence are difficult to evaluate. Although loaded with complicating factors, this report is from a credible source—a published paper by Dr. Dalton, author of the landmark work that first identified PMS.[15]

Once again, the differences between natural progesterone and the synthetic progestins must be addressed. If synthetic progestin is harmful for an adult, there is no question about its harm for a small, growing fetus. But, as emphasized, natural progesterone functions very differently, and your body produces huge quantities during pregnancy.

Contraception

Did you ever wonder why women who have had one ovary removed continue to ovulate every month? Didn't we assume that the ovaries took turns ovulating? Not exactly! After an egg is discharged, the progesterone buildup that occurs is responsible for sending a signal to the other ovary with a message that the egg-releasing is a *fait accomplis,* as indicated earlier. Progesterone is the messenger.

After ovulation, one of the results of the rapidly increasing progesterone levels is to make both the mucous linings and vaginal fluid thick and sticky enough to prevent additional sperm from entering the womb. (If the ovulation has resulted in fertilization, the egg will be up in the Fallopian tube near the ovary. The successful sperm will have entered the tube before progesterone buildup begins.) So natural progesterone may also be effective as a contraceptive. I'm not suggesting that you rely on this method to prevent pregnancy. Just be aware that progesterone supplementation before ovulation—if present in high doses—may have this contraceptive effect.[16] If you want to become pregnant and you are using natural progesterone to alleviate PMS symptoms, administer your natural progesterone on days 14 to 26 of your cycle—after ovulation.

Fertility

Although used in large amounts in synthetic forms for contraception, natural progesterone triggers fertility in human spermatozoa, suggesting a clinical application in the treatment of the different techniques of assisted fertilization.[17] In other words, it helps to normalize out-of-order conception functions. Natural progesterone can correct a luteal phase defect and result in an improved conception rate.[18] Note the suggestion for use during Days 14 to 26 following ovulation.

Increased Sex Drive

I have already related the appealing story of the remote group of island people who consume large quantities of a tuber similar to the Mexican yam. The libido rate of these people is extraordinarily high, yet their population rate is surprisingly low. Perhaps this is the quintessential story that demonstrates both the love-making *and* the contraceptive propensities of progesterone. (To protect this island against a population explosion, it will remain unidentified! For those who insist on following through, check the October 1992 issue of *National Geographic*.)[19]

American yams, by the way, do not have the same properties. Should you eat Mexican yams instead of applying the cream? They are not especially edible, and, because of nutrient-depleted soil and nutrient-depleting marketing delays (the time it takes to get food like Mexican yams from the garden to your table), my advice is to consider the transdermal cream.

Asthma

Premenstrual asthma flare-up is a well known phenomenon which may be remedied with progesterone.[20]

Epilepsy

Dr. Dalton offers this encouraging information for epileptics: "One of the most satisfying experiences is to diagnose and treat a woman with premenstrual epilepsy. She can be treated with progesterone and freed from all anticonvulsant tablets with their many unpleasant side effects."[21] A more recent report confirms Dr. Dalton's conclusions: "Natural progesterone and other antiestrogenic agents constitute rational and effective adjuncts to epilepsy therapy."[22] An even later study indicates that progesterone has an effect on epileptic seizure because of its barbiturate-like mechanism of action on brain metabolites.[23]

Prostate Cancer

Why include information about prostate cancer in a book *for and about* women? With the increasing incidence of prostate problems, why not be informed! If your "significant other" isn't a male, what about your father, brother, cousin, or friend? Here's the story: If a man has testicles removed as a result of prostate cancer, or has an undescended testicle as a result of DES used by his mother during pregnancy, loss of testosterone may lead to osteoporosis. This may be prevented or treated with natural progesterone. Natural progesterone has no feminizing effects and will accomplish the same bone-building benefits as testosterone.[24]

Teenage Acne

We have heard excellent reports of teenage acne clearing quickly with the use of natural progesterone cream.

Endometrial Hyperplasia

Endometrial hyperplasia (abnormal growth of cells in the mucous lining of the uterus) may develop because of estrogen use or estrogen invasion from the envrionment. Women may revert to normal endometrium when placed on natural progesterone.[25]

Hypertension
Research relating menopause and sex hormones to blood pressure concludes that natural progesterone is a protective factor for hypertension.[26] Synthetic progestins and estrogens, however, have been associated with increased sodium content of body cells, leading to hypertension.[27]

Skin Care
Dr. Atkins is especially enthusiastic about natural progesterone cream for skin care. He endorses its use because he finds it to be an exceptional wrinkle eradicator.[28] Many women report improved skin conditions, and the disappearance of hormone-related brown spots.

Cysts and Fibroids
Similar testimonials can be found regarding natural progesterone's effectiveness against polycystic breast disease (formation of many cysts) and cervical dysplasia (abnormal development of the cervix). These are potentially very serious conditions which require treatment plans directed by your physician. Reports with the use of progesterone, however, have been exciting, to say the least. (See page 253.) Within a short period of time, women have been giving accounts of seeing and feeling their fatty tumors breaking up.

Hormone-related Migraines
Accounts are streaming in about joint pain alleviation. Several women reported that the amount of cream in their jars was mysteriously disappearing, only to discover their husbands were the culprits. The men were "dipping in," based on the women's stories of pain relief success. (Progesterone is not a secondary sex hormone. Despite its special attibutes, it is neither male nor female in effect.)

Breast-Size Enhancement

In 1786, an English surgeon became the first to demonstrate that castration caused sex accessory tissues to shrink. But it wasn't until the 1930s that anyone discovered why this happened. Investigators at the University of Chicago noted that removing testes shut down production of testosterone, but when testosterone was injected back into castrated animals, these tissues were restored to normal size and function. A few women have reported an increase in breast size with the use of progesterone cream. Could the application of progesterone contribute to a "normalizing" consequence? (See Afterword, page 245.)

Researcher Beware!

As my research on natural progesterone progresses, I cannot help but be impressed with its positive results—clinically and in the laboratory. Occasionally, exceptions surface, but after careful examination of the studies, it becomes obvious that certain factions in our money-driven society don't want women to replace a risk-laden expensive drug with an inexpensive nonprescription and safer product.

The conclusions of one study, for example, looked at bone mineral responses *after* participants spent a year on estradiol, and then again a year later after the use of micronized progesterone.[29] (The process of micronizing reduces progesterone to finer particles for easier absorption.) Since the bone benefit observed was no different after the second year, it was determined that progesterone had no effect. Graphs presented in the study, however, show that the mineral density of some bones tested *did actually increase*. Physicians noting this study may be unaware of all the facts. Be a careful researcher! Don't pay attention to conclusions that result from drug-industry hype.

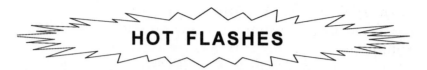

HOT FLASHES

➤ The transdermal route of hormone application may result in fewer adverse liver effects.
Jnl of Clinical Endocrinology and Metabolism, 1991.[30]

➤ Transdermal therapy represents an important advance in hormone therapy.
Drugs, 1990[31]

➤ The risk of cancer in long-term perimeno-pausal treatment with estrogen is not prevented by the addition of progestins—especially after a few years.
New England Jnl of Medicine, 1989[32]

➤ The risk of cancer with long-term perimeno-pausal estrogen treatment may be increased with the addition of progestins.
New England Jnl of Medicine, 1989[33]

➤ Natural progesterone helps to prevent the possible negative effects resulting from pituitary dysfunction.
Human Reproduction, 1992[34]

➤ Failure of current double-blind trials to relieve PMS with progesterone use is caused by using low-dose synthetic progestins.
Medical Hypotheses, 1990[35]

➤ Using natural progesterone as a contraceptive adds a new measure of safety for breast-feeding mothers, since the amount of the steroid secreted in mother's milk is not effectively absorbed by the infant.[36]
Jml of Steroid Biochem and Molecular Bio, 1991

➤ Women whose pregnancies end in miscarriages tend to have lower concentrations of progesterone.
Fertility and Sterility, 1993[37]

➤ Progesterone supplementation may affect pregnancy rates of in-vitro fertilization by increasing endometrial thickness, thereby enhancing receptivity for implantation.
Human Reproduction, 1992[38]

➢ A dose of 0.8-mg of the progestin *ST 1435* administered transdermally once a day appears to suppress ovulation.
Fertility and Sterility, 1992[39]

➢ Progesterone is essential for pregnancy.
Annals of Medicine, 1993[40]

➢ The normal monthly changes of female hormones can also affect the severity of responses to therapy in conditions such as asthma.
Jnl of the American Medical Womens Association, 1993[41]

➢ The advantages of delivering drugs through the skin for systemic therapy have been widely recognized and represent a growing sector in drug development.
Annals of Medicine, 1993[42]

➢ Transdermal delivery of steroids is a rapidly expanding field. In various clinical situations where hormonal replacement therapy is needed, this route of administration is a real breakthrough—especially considering the relative toxicity of some steroids when given orally.
Annals of Medicine, 1993[43]

➢ Progesterone has been demonstrated to be a good candidate for transdermal delivery.
Annals of Medicine, 1993[44]

➢ Most of the harmful adverse effects of ERT have been related to the absence of progestational balance.
Drugs, 1990[45]

➢ During the past decade, several isolated reports have linked an increased incidence of breast cancer with the use of synthetic progestins.
Cancer, 1993[46]

UPDATES
Fertility & Sterility 1996 Apr;65(4):860-2
The daily vaginal administration of progesterone for 10 days allowed useful serum progesterone levels to be reached, especially after estrogen therapy, and induced clear secretory changes in the endometrium.

American College of Obstetricians and Gynecologists 1996
Fibroids, also called myomas, are noncancerous
growths that can be as small as a pea or as large as
a grapefruit. Estrogen seems to increase their growth.

1996 Medical Tribune News Service
The most common cause of painful sexual intercouse
is vaginal dryness.

Bone 1997 Jan;20(1):17-25
Progesterone stimulates proliferation and differentiation of osteoblast bone cells.

1996 Medical Tribune News Service
Nearly 80 percent of the world's population depends
on alternative approaches for primary medical care.

Obstetrics and Gynecology 1996;88:227-233
About 70 percent of American women using the inject-
able contraceptive Depo-provera discontinue use
within a year, primarily because of side effects: heavier
and more frequent menstrual bleeding, amenorrhea
(loss of menstruation), increased cramping, weight
gain, headaches, depression, and nervousness. The
report concludes, "Women in the study should have
been well-informed."

Lancet, 1994, Nov 12, Vol 344:1364
Lower-dose estrogen pills often contain more powerful progestins to inhibit ovulation and prevent irregular
bleeding. The researcher stated: "I think the future out-
look for women is grim. A well-functioning ovary is not
a health risk. Oral contraceptives, which are meant to
inhibit this production, can cause problems."

Lancet 1996;347:959
Merck & Co sent letters to physicians in the USA about
severe oesophagitis with its drug Fosomax, used to
treat osteoporosis.

~~ ENDNOTES ~~ *The fantasy continues...*

Even in our fantasy, it's not easy to disentangle the complexities of menstrual, menopausal, and aging disorders, now so commonplace in our society. All long-term consequences of growing older are more amenable to prevention than to cure. But prevention is easier said than done.

Keep in mind that synthetic estrogen therapy can stimulate the breast, create proliferative endometrium, cause salt and fluid retention, increase body fat, interfere with thyroid hormone, cause depression and headaches, increase blood clotting, diminish libido, impair blood-sugar control, cause decline of zinc and retention of copper, reduce oxygen levels in all cells, cause endometrial cancer, increase the risk of breast cancer, and slightly restrain osteoclasts.

Natural progesterone, on the other hand, helps to: protect against fibrocysts, maintain secretory endometrium, function as a natural diuretic, use fat for energy, stimulate thyroid hormone action. Natural progesterone is also a natural antidepressant. It can normalize blood clotting, restore libido, normalize blood sugar levels, normalize zinc and copper levels, restore proper cell oxygen levels, prevent endometrial cancer, contribute to the prevention of breast cancer, stimulate osteoblasts, is a precursor of normal cortisone synthesis, and is necessary for the survival of the embryo!

~~~

According to *Lancet* (1997;349:406) and the *Annals of Emerging Medicine* (1997;29:255), the *Physician's Desk Reference,* better known as the PDR, found in nearly every doctor's office, clinic, and hospital nursing station in the USA, may contain out-of-date and incomplete information of the management of drug overdoses.

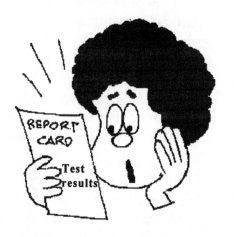

Tony, you failed your health test.
The four food groups are NOT
McDonald's, Kentucky Fried Chicken,
Dunkin' Doughnuts, and Pizza Hut!

15

CHOICES

HRT — YES OR NO ?

With all the information cited in these pages as background, we come full circle to the title of this book: *Hormone Replacement Therapy—Yes or No?* Let's review some of the facts.

In spite of all the proved disadvantages, the medical literature indicates that estrogen-progestin hormone replacement therapy has been confirmed as an effective prevention for osteoporosis and heart disease in postmenopausal women. But you are better informed now. It's still a tough decision, because hormone therapy involves judgment in order to weigh the pros and cons.

No one dies from vaginal atrophy, bladder dysfunction, or hot flashes. Quality of life and marriage, however, could be remarkably improved by relieving these symptomatic conditions with some form of hormone therapy.[1] Cancer, of course, is another matter.

After surveying current literature on hormone therapy in postmenopausal women, the medical journal *Family Practice* came to this less-than-satisfying conclusion: *Hormone therapies in postmenopausal women are controversial and provoke more questions than answers.*

The Nurses' Health Study revealed a 46-percent increase in ischemic stroke risk among nurses using estrogen replacement therapy, despite the fact that this group was comprised of women who had less diabetes, were non-smokers, and had less adiposity than those not using estrogen.[2]

Shouldn't the increased risk of breast cancer preclude the use of estrogen? How do we answer misleading reports that combinations of estrogen and progestins help to avoid uterine cancer? And what about the effects of *long-term* administration? Do the potential benefits of symptom relief justify the cost and treatment of large numbers of women who, without therapy, may never have developed complications attributable to lack of estrogen? Given these uncertainties, is postmenopausal administration of hormones reasonable or wise? The current literature does not provide adequate answers to these questions mainly because it generally does not consider natural progesterone as part of the protocol.[3]

Are physicians paying enough attention to the contraindications of HRT? According to generally accepted research, synthetic hormones should not be used for women who have had breast cancer, thrombophlebitis, hypertension, gallstones, diabetes, or undiagnosed abnormal genital bleeding.[4] If you or close members of your family are cancer-prone, you should be especially apprehensive about the relationship of postmenopausal use of estrogen and endometrial cancer.

Keep in mind that rates of endometrial cancer have risen sharply. Fluid retention, breast enlargement, and growth of preexisting uterine tumors have been noted. If these are familiar problems for you or close family members, estrogen therapy is contraindicated. Yet, as I lecture around the country, woman after woman tells me their physicians ignore these warnings—holding the false promise of bone and heart protection over their heads.

Breast tissue ages according to hormonal (primarily estrogen) exposure. Because of this fact and other similar variations studied internationally, *the incidence rates of breast cancer can actually be predicted throughout the world.*[5] Although association is not proof of cause, researchers are taking a hard look at these parallel statistics.

Estrogen therapy requires annual patient testing for blood-level evaluation (rather inaccurate testing at best). Urine and breasts need to be examined on a regular basis. Your physician is aware of the possibility of stimulating blood in urine, necessitating frequent checks. Women on long-term estrogen therapy have a 30-percent greater chance of developing breast cancer. Periodic endometrial biopsies for early detection of premalignant or malignant endometrial changes are recommended.[6] (Not to worry, says the doctor, we'll just perform a hysterectomy and remove the area that is symptomatic, which, needless to say, does nothing about getting to the cause!)

In making your decision, recall that estrogens do not restore lost bone and that withdrawal of estrogen therapy is followed by significant bone loss—suggesting that therapy must be ongoing for many years.[7] You become a patient—not only as long as you continue therapy, but also after you stop therapy. Even more depressing, the positive estrogen effects do not last more than three to five years.

As noted, several of the nutrition-oriented physicians I interviewed indicated that they prescribe very small amounts of estrogen *only if hot flashes and vaginal dryness are unbearable,* and for the rare osteoporotic patient for whom natural progesterone alone may not be sufficiently effective. These physicians are so concerned about estrogen therapy, they prescribe doses only to the point of making symptoms tolerable—but not necessarily to eliminate discomfort totally. Low-dose transdermal forms of less dangerous estrogens may avoid some complications of higher-dose oral therapy.[8]

CYCLIC ESTROGEN: ADDING PROGESTINS

Your physician may be influenced by tempting reports about reduced risks of estrogen therapy when progestins are added.[9] *Cyclic* estrogen administration prior to menopause is an effort to imitate nature. The patient uses progestin for ten days to initiate endometrial sloughing and then stops its use, but continues on estrogen the entire month. With this therapy, a woman may menstruate into her sixties and seventies. The disadvantage is the monthly withdrawal bleeding, and this would surely be considered a very serious side effect were it not for the fact that you've had your entire adult life to get used to menstruation. Whether or not this does actually reduce the risk of cancer is still debatable. But the handwriting is on the wall and it doesn't bode well.

A well-designed study to assess the side effects of medroxyprogesterone in replacement therapy warns: *Cyclic progestogen therapy appears to have preceded detailed evaluation of possible adverse side effects of progestogens.*[10] A warning that we have "jumped in" too soon!

When statements are made indicating that the combined therapy reduces risk, it is not clear whether the reduction is *to the level of* or *below* the risk observed in an untreated population. All progestins may cause physical, psychological, and metabolic side effects. In fact, side effects are common and there is a high incidence of bleeding in the first few months, which is unacceptable to many patients. (Once again—a reminder that progestins are synthetic, and differ from natural progesterone.)

The *FDA Consumer* discusses Depo-Provera, the quarterly contraceptive. Depo-Provera inhibits the production of another hormone, gonadotropin, which in turn, prevents ovulation. Depo-Provera also causes changes in the lining of the uterus that make pregnancy less likely. Note the following statements in this FDA-published journal:

➤ A link between Depo-Provera and breast cancer was first considered in the early 1970s in test animals. The studies were regarded as not applicable to humans. (Why not? The results of endless other similar studies are!)

➤ According to testimony presented to the *Fertility and Maternal Health Drugs Advisory Committee* of the FDA, trials demonstrating safety of the product were conducted in countries with breast cancer rates less than half that of the United States and therefore can't be accurately applied to women in this country.[11]

➤ Only three epidemiologic studies were done on Depo-Provera and breast cancer, and all three raised a red flag.[12]

➤ The bone density in 30 women who had been using Depo-Provera for at least five years was *less* than the bone density of other women of similar age.[13]

The FDA report noted that a professor with the Department of Obstetrics and Gynecology at the University of Southern California School of Medicine, said, "Oh, these women must have had preexisting tumors." (Arggghhhhh!!!) The National Women's Health Network disagrees with the benign conclusions of the researchers promoting Depo-Provera as safe.[14] What is Depo-Provera? *Synthetic progestin!*

Endometrial and breast cancer associated with continuous ERT were reported to be reduced with the use of cyclic progestins. More recent studies demonstrate this has not been the case. Again, the medical community jumped to conclusions before the drug had been used long enough for definitive, irrefutable evidence.[15] How do *you* feel about being a guinea pig?

SEQUENTIAL OR CONTINUOUS?

If you do decide on the prescribed replacement combination of estrogen plus synthetic progestin, the next question is: Should it be continuous or sequential? Some postmenopausal women receiving sequential treatment develop PMS-like symptoms when synthetic progestin is added.[16] Continuous combined estrogen and progestin preparations eliminate the inconvenience of regular progestin-induced withdrawal bleeding.[17] Any breakthrough bleeding occurring after a period of prolonged amenorrhea must be investigated by means of endometrial biopsy.[18] This makes you more than a participant—*you must become a patient.*

The continuous protocol has been eagerly embraced by women who don't want to be encumbered with the need to remember what day it is and when to take what. Many physicians, favoring compliancy, recommend what is easiest—*not necessarily what is good for your body.*

THE CHOICE

So when your doctor advocates estrogen treatment, you have a serious choice to make. You can agree to follow the advice, recognizing that when your hormones are being manipulated, you are handing over responsibility, which may be exactly what you want to do. Being the passive recipient of your doctor's choice of treatment may work for you. Not everyone wants to be in charge or make the changes. Or, you may want to be in control. Are you able to make the commitments necessary for the beneficial changes? Honest answers to these questions will help you to make the right personal decision. It's not always a matter of right or wrong. What you decide is going to be the best action for *you* is the important factor.

If you settle on a supplement-and-exercise regimen on your own, you make *yourself* accountable, so you need to be more earnest about lifestyle changes. It may take time before you are relieved of symptoms—unless you have been eating *whole, unprocessed food,* taking good *supplements,* and *exercising* routinely before the onset of menopause.

Have you considered yourself the victim of bad luck or bad genes? Or do you think you are among those whose genes are good enough to circumvent the hazards of our current environment? If you identify with the former, you should know that you *can* intercept heredity. Less than two percent of the world's population fits the latter category.

If you suffer from sweating and flushes, your choice may not be easy to come by. One of the benefits of estrogen is a quick relief of hot flashes. Estrogen can make a difference in your sleep. When you are exhausted from lack of sleep, the benefit of a restful night can be a powerful influence. The research is convincing, indicating that not only is symptomatic relief (from sweating episodes, sleep disturbance and hot flushes) observed during treatment, but that there are also improvements in terms of energy and emotions. Improvement in well-being, anxiety, depression, vitality, health, and self-control are supposed to take place, and women are told they will experience less tension and more satisfaction.[19,20]

Any of these benefits—if they are in fact realized—are short-lived at best.

Can these advantages be achieved another way, thereby eliminating the side effects of the usual HRT? I firmly believe that they can!

But what about the synthetic hormones and reduced risk of death from heart disease? *Studies show that the same protective effect supposedly provided by hormone therapy is seen in women who experience natural menopause—* without the use of hormone therapy! This was the conclusion after research on the reduction of cardiovascular disease-related mortality among postmenopausal women who use hormones, reported in the *American Journal of Obstetrics and Gynecology.*[21] Many more studies have shed new light on the therapy/reduced heart-disease risk correlations. (See the Afterword chapter.)

Again: risks associated with estrogen therapy relate to length of use. The apparent latent period is three to six years, after which problems increase rapidly.

Regardless of your decision, there are positive steps you can take to mitigate the potential dangers of estrogen therapy or the hazards of increased fractures, already outlined in previous pages.

Although so many practitioners and their patients acclaim the benefits of natural progesterone, too many are not getting this message. A brand-new indictment and analysis of medical practices, written by a physician (M. Konner, *Medicine at Crossroads*), still refers to progesterone only as the *pregnancy hormone.*[22] And too many other references in our latest journals describe the symptoms we have been discussing as "emotional."

CHINESE MEDICINE AND HERBOLOGY

In this era of interest in Eastern medicine and the use of herbs, I would be remiss not to mention Chinese medicine and herbology. Dr. Herb Kandel, a licensed acupuncturist and doctor of Oriental medicine who practices in Santa Maria, California, contributed the following information:

"Herbs can improve overall health as well as reduce common menopausal symptoms. Generally speaking, herbs are gentle on the body for two reasons: they are absorbed more slowly than single chemical extracts or synthetic pharmaceutical drugs; and constituents in herbs have multiple ingredients which are often counterbalancing to the active ingredients in that herb. The complex nature of herbal medicines may also explain certain herbs' ability to have self-regulating effects on the body. For example, the Chinese herb Dang Gui (Angelica sinensis) has properties which can both constrict an overly relaxed uterus and soften a cramping uterus. This ability to have multiple properties and thus help the body self-regulate is even more prominent in well-formulated herbal combinations.

"Three factors can help you to choose herbs wisely: 1) an understanding of the qualities, actions, and common uses of each herb; 2) any potential adverse effects of each herb; and 3) knowledge of your own body's strengths, weaknesses and particular needs. Information on herbs that have proved to be useful during menopause and for PMS follows.

"*Chaste Berries or Vitex (Agnus castus).* Vitex is the single most important western herb for regulating the period and reducing menopausal distress. Vitex stimulates the pituitary and helps the body produce progesterone. This herb has a balancing effect on estrogens while favoring progesterone. It is useful before menopause to normalize periods for as long as possible, as well as to treat painful periods. It is also effective in treating various problems associated with menopause.

"*Dang Gui (Angelica sinensis).* Dang Gui is a primary herb in Chinese medicine for treating menstrual irregularities, including delayed menses, pain during menstruation, and fatigue due to blood loss or deficiency. It has been adopted more widely in the west to treat menopausal syndromes but should not be used if excessive bleeding is present. It has a normalizing effect on muscles of the uterus, increases liver metabolism, reduces atherosclerosis in arteries (animal studies) and has proved effective for various pain syndromes. Studies do not demonstrate an estrogenic effect as has been reported by some. In fact, clinical evidence points to progesterone production, since women who take this herb alone in a dose too high often report midcycle bleeding and light-headedness or grogginess. It is best taken in a formula or with professional guidance. Dang Gui can also be added to soups. The western relative of Dang Gui, Angelica archangelica, often called *angelica*, has fewer antispasmodic properties. It is not generally indicated for menopause and is contraindicated during pregnancy.

"*Black Cohosh (Cimicifuga racemosa).* Black cohosh is very high in potassium and has a vasodilatory effect. Benefits include anti-inflammation and gentle sedation. Useful for menstrual pains and for reducing hot flashes, this herb lowers blood pressure and relaxes the muscles, as shown in animal studies. In Chinese medicine, it is used for swelling in the mouth, such as canker sores and swollen or painful gums, and for the early stage of measles. Some physicians warn that Black Cohosh is specifically estrogenic, and therefore, unopposed with progesterone, risks endometrial buildup. If taken for a prolonged period of time, it should be used in a well-rounded formula with other herbs.

"*Siberian Ginseng (Eleutherococcus senticosus).* This herb is a member of the ginseng family, with distinctively different effects from panax ginseng. Siberian ginseng is useful for increasing energy level and promoting enhanced tolerance to stress [as described more fully in Betty Kamen's booklet, *Siberian Ginseng: Up-to-Date Research on the Fabled Tonic Herb*]. It is useful for menopausal women who suffer from chronic fatigue or illness, frequent colds or flus, and sensitivity to emotional and environmental stress. Siberian ginseng must be taken on an ongoing basis for several weeks to notice the effects. Most women report feeling more resilient at an appropriate dose, or restless with increased irritability if the dose is too high. Here is one herb that can be taken safely as an individual herb. Product concentrations vary; start with the lowest recommended dose and adjust according to how you feel. Note: Panax Ginseng should be avoided for most women during menopause, as should Korean ginseng, which can elevate blood pressure and may increase endometrial build up. [Disregard literature indicating that women shouldn't take ginseng, and keep all of these facts in mind—especially concerning the advantages of Siberian ginseng.]

"*Herbs for Nervous Tension and Insomnia.* Catnip, chamomile, passion flower, lemon balm, and hops are all gentle herbs which can be used to promote calmness and improve sleep. These herbs can be steeped in tea (low dose) on a regular basis over a long period of time. They are widely available as tea blends or as loose tea in health food stores. Valerian root has stronger sedative properties and can be used temporarily for particularly stressful times, but should not be used consistently over a long period. Valerian and skullcap can be useful in the process of withdrawal from drugs or alcohol.

"Advice for all herbal sedatives: avoid habituation, use sedatives in combination for more effectiveness, use herbs to reinforce natural cycles of rest (after work, before bed), and avoid use during pregnancy.

"It is best to consult a trained practitioner when choosing to use Chinese herbal formulas for menopausal symptoms. The following, however, are Chinese herbs which can be added safely to soups or stews.

"*Cooked Rehmannia (Rehmanniae glutinosae).* Traditional indications: replenishes blood and essence; relieves weakness, fatigue, dryness, anemia, irregular uterine bleeding, dizziness; strengthens bones and marrow; moistens tissues. This herb is rich in oils containing essential fatty acids.

"*Cornus (Cornus officinalis).* Traditional indications: stabilizes 'kidney essence'; checks excessive sweating; strengthens bones and tendons; relieves frequent urination, dizziness, and excessive menstrual flow; enhances libido and fertility; strengthens low back and knee weakness.

"*Peony (Paeoniae lactiflorae).* Traditional indications: nourishes the blood and calms the liver; indicated for menstrual dysfunction, uterine bleeding, pain (especially spasms, cramps, or abdominal pain), night sweats, edginess, irritability, and mood swings.

"So you see that herbal and Chinese medicines can be useful in helping women journey through menopause in a more comfortable and self-empowered manner."

Herb Kandel, Santa Maria, California

We are grateful to Dr. Kandel for his vast experience and insights, and, especially, for his generous contribution.

HOMEOPATHY

Dr. Martin Milner, naturopathic physician of Portland, Oregon, provides information on homeopathy. Dr. Milner informs us that "homeopathy has successfully treated the symptoms of menopause for years. Constitutional homeopathic physicians commonly use a small selected group of remedies that effectively treat these symptoms. After symptoms are determined, the proper individualized remedy is given. The most commonly used remedies include Graphites and Sepia, followed by Sabina, Sanguinaria, and, to a lesser extent, Sarsparilla."

Following are Dr. Milner's specific suggestions for explicit problems.

➤ The mood swings and pelvic or uterine weakness of menopause often respond to Sepia.

➤ Night aggravations of symptoms in a relatively robust, fair-complexioned female often respond to Graphites.

➤ Sabina has a specificity action on the uterus itself, helping to heal the organ if involved with fibroids or abnormal menstrual flow patterns before menopause.

➤ The hot flashes of menopause often respond best to Sanguinaria.

➤ Urinary incontinence often associated with menopause resolves with Sarsaparilla.

For further assistance, contact a local homeopathic physician, or Dr. Martin Milner at the Center for Natural Medicine, Inc., Portland, Oregon 97214 (1-503-232-1100). Or, try Dr. Milner's Web Site: cnm-inc.com.

THE WANING EFFECT OF POSTMENOPAUSAL ESTROGEN THERAPY ON OSTEOPOROSIS

The October 14, 1993 issue of the *New England Journal of Medicine* published as its lead article the results of research demonstrating the waning effect of postmenopausal estrogen therapy on osteoporosis. The article reminds us that almost all physicians and their patients believe that estrogen treatment can prevent osteoporosis. What we now know, however, is that in women more than 75 years old, there is little difference in bone density between those who have taken estrogen and those who have not. The average age of hip fracture among postmenopausal women is 80 years! (Later studies support these results. See *Afterword*, page 245.)

The researchers conclude that ERT in the first decade after menopause cannot be expected to protect against osteoporotic fractures years later. They also validate what has been stated in earlier chapters here: the reduction in risk of hip fracture associated with estrogen treatment dissipates after treatment is stopped. *Estrogen treatment for 5 to 10 years soon after menopause is unlikely to preserve bone density or to prevent fractures in old age.*

The researchers suggest an alternative to the current trend of "estrogenizing" all women: "Start estrogen after osteoporotic fracture, an effective strategy that targets easily identified women who have a high risk of recurrent fracture and are likely to comply with treatment....Another alternative is to start estrogen treatment many years after menopause....Other effects of estrogen treatment should be considered...including a possible increase in the risk of breast cancer." *They still don't recognize the advantages of eliminating the synthetics and substituting the natural.*

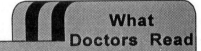

MEMOS

What Doctors Read

One way to understand what doctors are thinking is to look at what they are reading. Despite controversy and side effects, the following messages appeared in recent issues of prestigious medical journals. This is what your doctors write and read. What do you think?

➢ "Replacement therapy is the *assignment* of the gynecologist in order to protect the skeletal system."[23]

➢ "An enhanced tendency to exhaustion in menopause is dependent on *psychosocial* factors that correspond to a typically 'feminine' role enactment."[24]

➢ "Menopause is a medical condition; *natural approaches to menopause are less preferable;* women should take ERT for hot flashes. An educational approach could influence women's willingness to take ERT."[25]

➢ "*All* women should be followed by a gynecologist."

The practice of treating women as they go through one of life's most natural phases is now referred to as the emerging field of *menopause medicine*. My view? Menopause is a natural rite of passage and should not be treated as a disease!

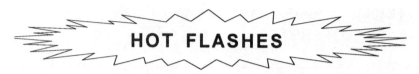

HOT FLASHES

➤ Overwhelming evidence shows that breast cancer risk is closely related to exposure to synthetic estrogens and progestogens.

Monograph, National Cancer Institute, 1994[26]

➤ [Synthetic] estrogen and progestin therapy have an adverse effect on bone because of their impact on magnesium excretion..

Magnesium and Trace Elements, 1991-92[27]

➤ Prenatal exposure to androgen-based synthetic progestin exerts a masculinizing and/or defeminizing influence on human behavior.

Psychoneuroendocrinology, 1991[28]

➤ Major compliance problems of replacement therapy include weight gain, resumption of withdrawal bleeding, and breast or endometrial cancer.

International Jnl of Clinical Pharmacology, Therapy, and Toxicology, 1992[29]

➤ Cessation of estrogen therapy restores bone loss.

Jnl of Obstetrics and Gynecology, 1992[30]

➤ Among the drawbacks of ERT are serious metabolic disturbances, particularly after oral administration of estrogens.

Annals of Medicine, 1993[31]

➤ Progestogens suppress the immune system.

Cleveland Clinical Journal of Medicine, 1994[32]

➤ Hormone replacement therapy decreases bone mineral density.

Maturitas, 1993[33]

➤ Progestogen may result in the return of menses.

Jnl of Obstetrics and Gynecology, 1992[34]

➤ Estrogens are implicated in breast and endometrial cancer. Synthetic progestens can cause some estrogen-like effects and some formulations place women at greater risk of having breast cancer.

Cancer, 1993[35]

➤ The long-term effect of postmenopausal estrogen therapy on bone density is not known.
New England Jnl of Medicine, 1993[36]

➤ Estrogen therapy becomes increasingly irrelevant as women approach the age at which the risk of fracture is highest.
New England Jnl of Medicine, 1993[37]

➤ There are estrogen-dependent and age-dependent components of bone loss. By the age of 70, the age-dependent component predominates.
Jml of Clinical Endocrin & Metabolism, 1990[38]

➤ Five or even 10 years of early postmenopausal estrogen therapy would have a trivial residual effect on bone mineral density at age 75.
Bone Mineral, 1990[39]

IN CONCLUSION ~

~ the positive benefits I have heard from coast to coast surpassed any expectations. Typical comments follow.

"I never knew I could feel this good."

"No more Prozac. I am calm, cool, and collected."

"My vaginal dryness is a problem of the past."

"I didn't know anything was wrong with me until I started applying this cream."

"Ever since my wife has been on the cream, I am a better driver."

"I have been able to feel and see my fatty tumors break up and disappear."

"For the first time in five years, I have ventured out. My panic disorder is gone."

"No more breast tenderness. For the first time in years, I could touch this area without discomfort."

"No more arthritic pain!"

"At last! A good night's sleep!"

"I can't believe it! No migraine in months."

"My husband makes sure I am never without this panacea that changed my life (and his, too!)."

~~ ENDNOTES ~~ *From fantasy to reality!*

Twenty-three percent of hospitalization is iatrogenic— caused by a doctor. It is no wonder that a survey published in *New England Journal of Medicine* indicates that *unconventional medical help is sought by at least one-third of the United States population.* Americans made 425 million visits to such providers in 1990—compared with 388 million visits to all family doctors, internists, and other primary care physicians combined.

According to the report, patients rarely tell their physicians of their extracurricular unorthodox medical ventures. Three-quarters of the money spent is out of their own pockets and is not reimbursed by insurance companies. Unorthodox therapies are those that are not usually taught at medical schools or practiced in hospitals. The people most likely to use such therapy are well-educated, middle-income folk.

Dr. Joe Jacobs, director of the National Institutes of Health's Office of Alternative Medicine, said the popularity of alternative medicine demonstrates a hunger among Americans for more humane and less invasive treatments than those ordinarily practiced by standard doctors. Jacobs was most disturbed by the finding that 72 percent of those using unconventional therapies did not bother telling their doctors. "Some of these alternative therapies take a holistic and more caring view of a patient," he said.[40]

So we ask the question again: Should you treat yourself with natural progesterone?

I'm lucky. I don't have to answer the question of whether or not to apply natural progesterone cream for myself because I have access to a number of physicians who think the way I do about nutrition, lifestyle, and health. In other words, not only do I go to a doctor I can trust, but my physician cooperates with me and even advocates many of the new and sometimes unconventional approaches that I believe are best. So my choice is easy.

But what if your doctor is less agreeable? What if your doctor is more conservative, isn't aware of the latest findings in this area, doesn't respond well to suggestions from a patient, or is antagonistic to the use of natural progesterone or any other treatment you may decide to use?

It would be easy for me to simply say, "Find another doctor." This is not practical advice for many. You may not have *any* physician whom you can see regularly, let alone easy access to an *acceptable* one. Finding a specialist who will work with you on a treatment regimen considered unorthodox may be out of the question.

Ultimately, we all have to be our own doctors. What you eat and how you live contributes far more to your long-term health than anything a medical doctor will ever be able to do for you. Of course there are obvious exceptions, where major interventions are lifesaving. I think you get the point. The responsibility for good health is primarily your own. Hopefully, you'll act *before* you begin to notice the first faint rumblings of trouble.

Specific advice? Know your body as well as you possibly can and do what *you* believe is best. Even if your physician is downright hostile to the use of natural progesterone or any other treatment you may decide to use, don't cut off communications. Keep your doctor informed of your personal health decisions and their results, if you possibly can. The flow of information will help to give us all the knowledge to stay healthy.

AFTERWORD
1997 Update
Testimonials

Stories crediting natural progesterone for positive benefits have been streaming my way. Those familiar with my work know that I don't usually cite anecdotes, but rather well-conducted studies published in prestigious journals. I report these accounts, however, because I personally know and trust the sources. I can't help but believe that this kind of information will find its way into our conservative medical community in due time. (The studies are, in fact, beginning to surface.) Here are a few of the stories:

An interesting "side effect" came from my own daughter. "Mom," she said, "I need to get new bras. I am one cup-size larger. I know it's the progesterone!" My daughter, a grown woman and mother herself, is not one to come to frivolous or unfounded conclusions. So I checked with the MD clinicians and discovered that, in some women, the use of natural progesterone cream can cause an increase in breast size as it attempts to normalize hormone ratios. Ladies, don't expect a Marilyn Monroe outcome, but for those who would like a normalizing mammary gland increase, this may be a risk-free alternative.

My son's internist, a woman with a 20-year-old daughter, remarried at age 45. Her new husband, ten years younger, wanted a child. After conceiving with much difficulty, followed by two miscarriages, this physician started applying natural progesterone cream. After one month of application, she conceived without delay (at age 47) and experienced a normal pregnancy, an easy delivery, and a healthy baby.

Pat Kinney, a 67-year-old psychotherapist in Woodmere, New York, was told she had signs of bone density loss. She used natural progesterone cream for one year, and returned for testing. *Her bone condition had improved.* Her doctor remained impassive when she told him what she had been doing. "Isn't it unusual to show improvement at my age?" asked Pat. Her doctor simply didn't respond.

Beth Hirsch, 36, of New York City, said, "Tests showed I had virtually no progesterone. When I started using natural progesterone cream, my poor sleep problems, along with my miserable fatigue and debilitating migraines, all disappeared."

Valerie Donigan, cohost of the Donigan Nutrition hour in Boca Raton, Florida, thought she would be enslaved to a lifetime of overweight and infertility. She had a long history of anovulatory cycles and amenorrhea. Obsessive exercise habits and unhealthful dieting did nothing to control her weight. Valerie finally made the connection between lack of progesterone and thyroid function. She introduced nutrients (selenium, zinc, copper, and a thyroid glandular) plus natural progesterone cream. Her energy levels rose to new heights as pounds dropped off and her body temperature rose to normal. She gradually came off the thyroid supplementation but maintained the natural progesterone application (and her low weight). In her effort to become pregnant and have 28-day cycles, she increased the potency of the cream. She enjoyed a healthy pregnancy—once assumed to be something she could never experience—and is the proud mother of a very healthy and beautiful baby girl.

Laurel Endrin of Salt Lake City, Utah, is lucky. She has been using progesterone cream for twelve years, recommended by her physician to treat her endometriosis. She had been totally free of PMS after use of the cream, and now smiles in silence as she listens to her friends complain of menopausal symptoms. *Laurel is symptom-free.*

Donna Mulaney of Chevy Chase, MD, confronted her physician when she became empowered with information. "Why haven't you ever checked my progesterone levels?" she asked. After stammering a bit, her physician said, "Let's do it now." "You can't do it now," she responded. "I'm in my luteal phase." (Progesterone peaks in the luteal phase of the cycle.)

Donna Ragsdale, host of a nutrition program in High Point, North Carolina, said, "Betty, I can't even count the many women who heard you on my show and have since reported incredible results with the use of the natural progesterone cream."

Trudy Harris, 28, of Midland, Michigan, reported: "My mom had been using natural progesterone cream successfully for menopausal symptoms. She finally persuaded me to try it for my PMS. Now my cycle starts without any pre-announcements!"

Rose Lebow of Wichita, Kansas, used progesterone cream to shrink a large grapefruit-sized uterine fibroid tumor. Mission totally successful in four months! (See page 252.)

Frequently Asked Questions

Won't HRT protect my heart? My doctor says it will!

Many women are encouraged to take synthetic hormones because of heart-protective reports. A team of Dutch epidemiologists set the record straight. Researchers from Leiden University Hospital in the Netherlands analyzed 18 large HRT studies, comparing the risk of heart disease with risk of cancer. They showed that the same studies indicating that HRT protected against heart disease also demonstrated low rates of cancer. In fact, the greatest reduction in heart disease correlated with the largest decrease in cancer. But, according to this report, editorialized in the *Harvard Health Letter*, HRT does NOT protect against cancer. Endless accepted research validates the increased risk of cancer with the use of HRT. There is no question that women who take HRT have a *higher* risk of developing cancer. The researchers concluded that the women used in these studies were healthier than nonusers of HRT and had a lower risk of heart disease in the first place. Other epidemiologists confirm these results.[1] Please don't be taken in by the heart-disease scare! (Read more on the subject on pages 1 and 2.)

Can I improve my hormones by changing my diet?

Yes, and here's just one example: As the intake of soy foods rise, the weak estrogenic activity of plant phytoestrogens may reach biologically effective levels, having an estriol-like effect. The active ingredients are *isoflavones*. Tofu has the highest content (perhaps because of the fermentation process), soy drinks contain lesser amounts, and soy-based formulas are usually devoid of isoflavones.[2] (See soy caveat on page 73.)

I'm 40. Can the doctors tell me *now* if I'm going to be a candidate for osteoporosis?

Here are some of the many early predictors of osteoporosis:

~ Meat eaters are more vulnerable. Vegetarians are less likely to suffer from this disease. (See page 155.)

~ Those with prematurely gray hair (50% gray by age 40) are much more likely to have osteoporosis. The earlier you gray, the higher the risk. In normal white populations, graying starts at an average age of 34, and 50% of the population is 50% gray at age 50. (By contrast, blacks do not gray until 10 years later.)[3]

~ Anecdotal evidence of a link between excess alveolar bone resorption in the mandible and osteoporosis has been validated by several studies. (See page 138.) Women with low bone density have fewer teeth. In fact, women with severe postmenopausal osteoporosis are 3 times more likely to have no teeth than their normal counterparts.[4]

Supported by grants from the Public Health Service, risk factors for hip fracture in 10,000 women were studied and reported in the March 25, 1995 issue of *New England Journal of Medicine.* Guess what? We could have saved the taxpayers all that money. Researchers concluded that you are at greater risk if:

~ You drink coffee. (Risk increases with amount. See page 139.)

~ You spend fewer than four hours a day on your feet. (Weight-bearing exercise helps strengthen bone. See page 152.)

~ You can't rise from a chair without using your arms.

~ Your vision is poor or you have poor depth perception. (You will be more inclined to fall frequently.)

~ You take antidepressant drugs. (These medications increase the risk of falling.)

~ You smoke. (Current smokers have about twice the risk as nonsmokers or former smokers. See page 72.)

~ You are in poor health .

~ You have a history of maternal hip fracture. (Do we inherit physical propensities or do we inherit diets?)

~ You weigh the same or less at menopause than at age 25. The more weight gained since age 25, the lower the risk.

~ Risk decreases with increasing numbers of births.

~ Dietary calcium is not related to risk of hip fracture, even at very low intake. (I love this last one! What have I been saying all along?)

The researchers tried to excuse the fact that their studies showed no correlations between estrogen therapy and protection against hip fractures by stating that women who are on ERT are more likely to have severe osteoporosis to begin with. This flies in the face of the current trend of prescribing estrogen therapy to each and every woman, regardless of bone status.[5] It also contradicts research that shows that women who seek help from physicians are usually more health-minded. Are they catching at straws looking for excuses for results they don't like?

So if my hair turned gray early, I've had trouble with my teeth, I eat meat daily, drink coffee, etc., etc., is it too late to protect my bones?
Of course not! It's never too late to improve your health. Note all the references to progesterone and how its application can help to build bone back—even in very senior women.

Can progesterone help PMS and muscle cramping?
Progesterone is a good *antispastic*. If you have low levels of progesterone or magnesium you may suffer spasms in your temples as well as in your uterus because this impacts on smooth muscle. Rubbing the cream on your temples or pubic area could help your PMS migraine or uterine spasms. Once the migraine or uterine spasm is under way, this remedy won't help. So massage at first sign of a problem.

I've had breast cancer. Can I use progesterone cream?
A study published in *Fertility and Sterility* in 1995 demonstrated that an increased progesterone level—achieved by applying progesterone to the breast—significantly decreases breast-cell proliferation. Conclusions drawn from this research: Topically applied progesterone is well absorbed and will reduce the risk of breast cancer because of the decreased cell proliferation. Estrogen dominance, which promotes breast cancer, may be prevented with the use of natural progesterone cream.

Should men apply progesterone cream?

Progesterone may be prescribed for men who are deficient in testosterone because steroids help bone growth in men as well as women. Excess progesterone in males gets shunted into the testosterone pathway, which may be why men are reporting increased libido with use of the cream. (Purely anecdotal at this point in time, but extremely noteworthy: A chiropractor in Charlotte, North Carolina reported full return of libido following decline caused by high blood pressure medication.)

A new cream designed specifically for men has been released. In addition to progesterone and wild yam extract, it contains herbs known to help prevent and lessen prostate problems, such as saw palmetto, Siberian ginseng, and damiana.

What if I'm on birth control pills containing synthetic progestins?

All the more reason to use natural progesterone. Dr. Corsello insists that her patients on the Pill use natural progesterone— especially since synthetic progestins decrease your body's own production of natural progesterone.

Will using progesterone cream counteract the effect of my birth control pill?

Not at all. There is not enough progesterone in a well-designed product to produce the contraceptive effect.

Should women who miscarry be put on progesterone cream prior to conception?

Miscarriages have risen to one in four, and are still increasing. Studies point to progesterone deficiency as playing a major role in this outcome. The measurement of progesterone is used as a method of assessing reproduction status in some animals. Uterine bleeding in the second trimester, leading to abortion, is also related to low levels. Check with your OB/GYN about continuing the use of natural progesterone after conception.

Is it true that pollution is responsible for increased infertility?

An important article in *Lancet* should dispel any doubt about the power of our environment and our diets as they relate to sex hormones. Infertility has increased from 10 to 25 percent in recent years, and women are not alone in these statistics. The decline in sperm density and quality and semen volume from 1940 to 1990 has been significant and alarming. The incidence of testicular and prostate cancer has also increased during the same relatively short time period. Researchers report that such remarkable deterioration is due to environmental rather than genetic factors. Environmental chemicals that possess estrogenic activity are responsible for the increased frequency of reproductive abnormalities, just as reproductive changes in wildlife have been associated with environmental pollution. Exposure of the male fetus to high concentrations of estrogen compounds could be the triggering factor. Known as *xenoestrogens*, the defects they induce do not become apparent for 20 to 40 years. These estrogenic pollutants range from automobile exhaust, to pesticides like DDT to PCBs, to phthalates used in plastic wraps (yes, the kind we store food in, wear, sleep on, and sit on).[7] So here's further proof of the estrogenic contamination in our environment and the need for natural foods and progesterone to help put things in balance.

Is there a natural remedy for vaginal dryness?

The solution for this problem is vaginal application of natural progesterone cream, plus the vaginal insertion of a vitamin E soft-gel capsule. (See page 210.) This treatment is almost always effective. If, however, a more dramatic remedy is required, estriol cream (prescribed by your physician) may help, mainly because the lower 1/3 of the urethra is estriol-sensitive.

Can natural progesterone help ovarian cysts?

At the risk of repetition, natural progesterone cream can help ovarian cysts, PMS, fibrocystic mastitis, infertility, postpartum depression (which sets in just about the time that progesterone levels decrease), and more—mainly because these problems are related to estrogen excess.

What about DHEA? Should I be taking it?

DHEA has created quite a stir. (See page 41 for caveats.) It is somewhat similar to progesterone, but has its own distinctions. As indicated earlier, one of its functions is to make some of the estrogens. The chart on page 43 shows that both DHEA and progesterone are produced from pregnenolone. Consequently, it is also theorized that if enough DHEA is present, pregnenolone will be converted to progesterone (although DHEA does not convert *directly* to progesterone).

DHEA levels are significantly *higher* in PMS subjects around ovulation, as compared to controls. That doesn't mean it won't help if taken at other times of the month. If DHEA is working to alleviate PMS, etc., it may work this way: DHEA breaks down into a compound called 5-androstene-3B, 17B-diol. This compound binds to estrogen receptors. So, like the phytoestrogen foods that can also occupy these receptor sites, it may prevent estrogen overload, thereby indirectly promoting a healthier hormone balance. Keep in mind that it is contraindicated in those with blood sugar problems because of its negative effect on insulin resistance.

And then, sometimes, we borrow from Peter to pay Paul, and issues can be totally confusing. DHEA has been shown to reduce obesity in test animals. However, within the first years after menopause, moderate excess body weight significantly *reduces* vertebral postmenopausal bone loss.[8]

I heard something about applying the cream to spayed animals. What's the story?

Veterinarian Goeffrey Broderick of Huntington, New York, plans to apply the cream behind spayed animals' ears—a place they can't lick. Since dogs have no responsibilities (children, work, dinner, shopping, cooking, chauffeuring), they just lie down and sleep when they suffer the same symptoms as women whose ovaries have been removed or are hormonally unbalanced (mood shifts, etc.). The dogs become lazy and fat, but Dr. Broderick anticipates that his progesterone-treated dogs will be lively and healthy. (His experiment was delayed because his wife stole his first jar of cream. She is having such positive results, she refuses to share the bounty.)

I have fibroids. Can I use progesterone cream?
William C. Bryce, M.D., of Azusa, California, is among the many physicians recommending natural progesterone cream to his patients. He offers this information about uterine fibroid tumors: "Fibroids often cause or are coincidental with heavier periods, irregular bleeding, and/or painful periods. Due to their mass, they may cause a dropped uterus later in life when pelvic floor supports weaken, leading to urinary incontinence. The good news is that after menopause, fibroids routinely atrophy.

"Contemporary medical treatment is usually surgical, often re-sulting in hysterectomy. Fibroid tumors, like breast fibrocysts, are a product of estrogen dominance. Estrogen stimulates their growth and lack of estrogen causes them to atrophy. Estrogen dominance is a much greater problem than recognized by con-temporary medicine. Many women in their 30s begin to have anovulatory cycles. As they approach the decade before meno-pause, they are producing much less progesterone than expected but still produce normal (or more) estrogen. They retain water and salt, breasts swell and become fibrocystic, they gain weight (especially around the hips and torso), become depressed and lose libido, their bones suffer mineral loss, and they develop fibroids. All are signs of estrogen dominance, i.e., relative progesterone deficiency.

"When sufficient natural progesterone is replaced, fibroid tu-mors no longer grow in size (generally they decrease in size) and can be kept from growing until menopause after which they will atrophy. This is the effect of reversing estrogen dominance."

People are more nutrition-aware than ever before. Aren't fewer women succumbing to ERT?
An estimated 13.6 million prescriptions were dispensed for oral estrogens in 1982, *but the number jumped to 31.7 million in 1992.* Prescriptions for oral progestin increased from 2.3 million to 11.3 million in that same time period. Premarin is the most widely prescribed drug in the United States at this time. Its users top 10 million!

Why is progesterone, rather than estrogen, now considered the hormone of importance?

Progesterone is capable of transforming itself into estrogen and other adrenal steroids. (Adrenal steroids get used up during stress reactions). It also regulates many vital organ functions, including thyroid performance, glucose metabolism, and mineral mechanisms. When we are oversaturated with estrogen or estrogen-like substances (obtained from food or environmental pollutants and even from excessive growth of Candida albicans in the gut), we do not seem to be able to compensate with an adequate production of progesterone.

Why are we all so progesterone-deficient?

Contamination of our food supply, pollutants, poor gut ecological balance, poor nutrient status, excessive stress, and estrogen dominance are all contributing factors.

Can I use progesterone if I've just had a baby?

A major cause for postpartum depression is the reduced progesterone level that sets in about 6 to 10 weeks after delivery. Use of natural progesterone helps to prevent this event.

Is it true that progesterone can help my skin?

Menopause (and even PMS) leads to the acceleration of all aging processes throughout the body. The skin is a visible sign of aging, and internal organs are jeopardized as well. Get rid of the problems, and you help to "reverse" the aging process.

Do we understand how the herbs you mention help to balance our hormones?

Siberian ginseng, Dong Quai, and black cohosh are natural estrogen-mimicking substances. They help to block the re-uptake of estradiol—a villainous cancer-causing process—in the uterine lining and in breasts and ovaries. (See p. 233-237.)

If I must take estrogen, is there a safer form?

Not all estrogens are created equal. Estrone and estradiol have been implicated in many problems associated with estrogen therapy. Estriol, however, may exert protective functions.

I've had a hysterectomy. Can I use progesterone cream?
Since your hysterectomy has curtailed production of hormones (see page 237), the use of natural progesterone is highly recommended by nutrition-aware physicians. Besides, the hysterectomy eliminated the area of symptoms, but did not address the cause. The longer a woman is exposed to estrogen, unopposed by adequate amounts of natural progesterone, the higher the incidence of uterine and breast cancer.

Most women are told by their physicians that they MUST be on estrogen therapy if they've had hysterectomies. Just think of why you needed the hysterectomy. Large fibroids? Cysts? Endometriosis? Cancer? Wasn't it estrogen dominance that caused these problems to begin with?

The doctor rarely tells you that your ovaries will eventually curtail hormone production if you've had your uterus removed, or that your adrenal glands do the same if you've had your ovaries removed. As explained in these pages, you are still going to be exposed to exogenous sources of estrogen. Many women have reported success in slowly getting off estrogen while using a safe, natural progesterone source. Hysterectomy or no, synthetic estrogen is not in your best health interest.

Note: Sparing your ovaries and tying off the artery that supplies blood to them also affects their function.

Remind your doctor that hormone imbalance suggests that other functions are no doubt operating below par as well, and that you know about the use of safe herbs that work adaptogenically. (See page 113.)

If the cream doesn't seem to be working, does it mean I need something more powerful?
If you are not having success, you should see a physician. You may need a detoxification program. When cells are toxic, they have absorption difficulties. Other problems may be at hand, too, so please seek help from someone who understands the biochemistry and can help you achieve optimal health.

HOW TO USE THE FOOD TABLES

The food tables that follow list the calcium and phosphorous content of 157 common foods, silicon content of 73 fruits and vegetables, and boron content for 5 representative vegetables.

Use the calcium/phosphorous table to insure that your diet provides enough calcium, and to monitor the amount of phosphorous in comparison to calcium. Keep in mind that a natural diet—the diet that our bodies are designed to thrive on—contains only a little more phosphorous than calcium. Too much phosphorous in comparison to calcium interferes with incorporating new calcium into bone structure. Even if your bones are old, you need new calcium to make up for the calcium that is constantly being removed for use by other tissues.

There are 28 grams (g) in an ounce, so 100 g is about four ounces, or roughly a portion the size of your fist. A milligram (mg) is one one-thousandth of a g. The first calcium and phosphorus columns in the table are under the label "mg per 100 g." So if we had pure calcium, the table would indicate 100,000 mg per 100 g. A more typical value for vegetables, 100 mg per 100 g, means that the calcium content of the food is one part in one thousand, or one-tenth of a percent, by weight. Alfalfa sprouts, topping the list at 1,754 mg of calcium per 100 g of food, is 17.5 parts per thousand, or 1.75 percent calcium by weight.

The calcium and phosphorous columns on the right side of the table, under the label "mg per serving," might be more useful for menu planning. Here the amounts are corrected by the typical serving size, as indicated in the far right column.

You should include at least 1,000 mg of calcium in your diet every day. Don't be tempted to concentrate on dairy products (or even supplements). Absorption and assimilation of calcium from dairy sources are not as good as from grain and vegetable sources.

The "bad" and "good" columns of the table are useful for assessing the amount of phosphorous as compared to calcium.

Foods with more calcium (Ca) and less phosphorous (P) have a higher number under the "good" label. This number is simply the ratio of Ca-to-P. A higher number under "Ca/P" is a better food for helping your body maintain the proper Ca-to-P ratio. The "bad" column is the inverse ratio, P-to-Ca. A high number here works against you.

Take time to study the tables. Note that many foods associated with good nutrition have high numbers in the "bad" column. Garlic, for example, scores 7.0 bad points, and mushrooms, 11.3! It would be a mistake to avoid these foods because of this ratio. Fish doesn't look too good, either, but fish should be a major component of your diet (broiled or baked, not fried, please).

Use the table to find foods that supply needed calcium without increasing the phosphorus burden. Stand-out foods in the "good" column include cranberries, olives, and oranges. Kelp is an extremely valuable seasoning and can also assist in reducing sodium intake. Alfalfa is an unbeatable source of calcium without much phosphorous, and a number of other vegetables like collard leaves and Swiss chard have excellent Ca/P ratios.

The tables for silicon show the amount of this element, in mg per 100 g, for various fruits. No guideline is available for recommended daily intake, but it makes sense to give the foods that are high in silicon a special place on your shopping list. Dare I suggest "an apple a day..."?

Data for boron is hard to find, probably because the boron content of foods varies tremendously with the boron content of the soil in which it is grown. The tables show high and low values after testing several different samples of each food. The consequences of modern agriculture techniques result in less boron in foods than more traditional methods of farming. This is a negative health factor and one of the best arguments for buying organic produce from small farms. There is still no guarantee that the boron content will be sufficient, but at least by diversifying the sources of your food, you can improve the odds.

VEGETABLES	mg per 100 grams		P/Ca	Ca/P	mg per serving		serving
	calcium	phosph.	(bad)	(good)	calcium	phosph.	size
alfalfa	1754	251	0.1	7.0	1989	284	4 oz.
artichoke, cooked	51	69	1.4	0.7	58	78	4 oz.
asparagus, cooked	21	50	2.4	0.4	6	14	1 oz.
asparagus, uncooked	22	63	2.9	0.4	6	18	1 oz.
baked potatoes, with skin	9	65	7.2	0.1	20	147	8 oz.
beets, boiled	14	23	1.7	0.6	16	26	4 oz.
broccoli, cooked	88	62	0.7	1.4	100	70	4 oz.
Brussels sprouts, cooked	32	72	2.2	0.4	37	82	4 oz.
cabbage, cooked	130	230	1.8	0.6	147	261	4 oz.
carrots, raw	37	36	1.0	1.0	42	41	4 oz.
cauliflower, raw	25	56	2.2	0.4	28	64	4 oz.
celery, raw	39	28	0.7	1.4	44	32	4 oz.
chard	81	36	0.4	2.3	92	41	4 oz.
collard leaves & stems	203	82	0.4	2.5	230	93	4 oz.
corn, canned or cooked	4	48	12.0	0.1	5	54	4 oz.
cucumber, raw, unpeeled	26	28	1.1	0.9	29	32	4 oz.
dandelion greens	375	148	0.4	2.5	106	42	1 oz.
eggplant, steamed	11	26	2.4	0.4	13	30	4 oz.
French fried potatoes	15	111	7.4	0.1	34	251	8 oz.
garlic	29	202	7.0	0.1	8	57	1 oz.
green beans, cooked	50	37	0.7	1.3	57	42	4 oz.
green lima beans, raw	52	142	2.7	0.4	59	161	4 oz.
green peas, canned	20	66	3.3	0.3	23	75	4 oz.
green peas, fresh cooked	23	99	4.3	0.2	26	112	4 oz.
green peas, frozen	19	86	4.5	0.2	22	98	4 oz.
kale leaves	249	73	0.3	3.4	282	83	4 oz.
kidney beans	46	91	2.0	0.5	53	103	4 oz.
lettuce, iceberg	20	22	1.1	0.9	23	25	4 oz.
mung bean sprouts, raw	20	64	3.2	0.3	23	73	4 oz.
mushrooms, cooked or canned	6	68	11.3	0.1	7	77	4 oz.
onions, cooked	24	29	1.2	0.8	27	33	4 oz.
parsley, raw	204	63	0.3	3.2	58	18	1 oz.
pickles, dill or sour	26	21	0.8	1.2	29	24	4 oz.
potato, white	29	188	6.5	0.2	65	426	8 oz.
potato salad	19	63	3.3	0.3	22	72	4 oz.
romaine or leaf lettuce	68	25	0.4	2.7	77	28	4 oz.
sauerkraut, canned	36	18	0.5	2.0	41	20	4 oz.
spinach, steamed	93	38	0.4	2.4	105	43	4 oz.
squash, cooked	25	25	1.0	1.0	28	28	4 oz.
squash, uncooked	28	29	1.0	1.0	64	66	8 oz.
string beans	119	104	0.9	1.1	270	235	8 oz.
succotash, frozen	13	85	6.5	0.2	15	96	4 oz.
sweet potato, baked	40	58	1.5	0.7	91	132	8 oz.
sweet potato, candied	37	43	1.2	0.9	84	97	8 oz.
Swiss chard, steamed	73	24	0.3	3.1	83	27	4 oz.
tomato paste, canned	27	70	2.6	0.4	31	79	4 oz.
tomato puree, canned	13	34	2.7	0.4	29	77	8 oz.
tomato, canned	6	19	3.2	0.3	14	43	8 oz.
tomato, uncooked	13	27	2.1	0.5	15	31	4 oz.
vegetables, mixed frozen	29	74	2.5	0.4	33	83	4 oz.
yellow snap beans	56	43	0.8	1.3	64	49	4 oz.

GRAINS AND GRAIN PRODUCTS	mg per 100 grams		P/Ca	Ca/P	mg per serving		serving
	calcium	phosph.	(bad)	(good)	calcium	phosph.	size
bran flakes	53	358	6.8	0.1	60	405	4 oz.
brown rice, cooked	12	73	6.1	0.2	14	83	4 oz.
corn flakes	16	32	2.0	0.5	18	36	4 oz.
farina, instant	77	60	0.8	1.3	174	136	8 oz.
French bread	45	85	1.9	0.5	13	24	1 oz.
graham crackers	40	143	3.6	0.3	11	41	1 oz.
hamburger/hot dog buns	73	87	1.2	0.8	42	49	2 oz.
macaroni & cheese	181	161	0.9	1.1	410	365	8 oz.
oat meal, cooked	9	58	6.6	0.2	20	133	8 oz.
pancakes	220	338	1.5	0.7	499	766	8 oz.
pizza	221	195	0.9	1.1	502	442	8 oz.
pretzels	22	132	6.1	0.2	25	149	4 oz.
shredded wheat	43	389	9.1	0.1	49	441	4 oz.
spaghetti with meat sauce	50	95	1.9	0.5	113	216	8 oz.
toasted wheat germ	48	1085	22.7	0.0	54	1230	4 oz.
waffles	113	173	1.5	0.7	257	393	8 oz.
wheat bran	119	1121	9.4	0.1	135	1271	4 oz.
white bread, enriched	100	115	1.2	0.9	113	130	4 oz.
white rice, cooked	10	28	2.8	0.4	11	32	4 oz.
whole wheat flour	41	372	9.1	0.1	12	105	1 oz.

FRUITS	mg per 100 grams		P/Ca	Ca/P	mg per serving		serving
	calcium	phosph.	(bad)	(good)	calcium	phosph.	size
apples	7	10	1.4	0.7	16	23	8 oz.
apricots, dried	67	108	1.6	0.6	76	122	4 oz.
apricots, uncooked	17	34	2.0	0.5	19	38	4 oz.
avocado	10	42	4.1	0.2	23	96	8 oz.
banana	8	26	3.3	0.3	18	59	8 oz.
blueberries	15	13	0.9	1.2	17	15	4 oz.
cantaloupe	14	16	1.1	0.9	32	36	8 oz.
cherries	22	19	0.9	1.2	25	22	4 oz.
cranberries	124	20	0.2	6.2	140	23	4 oz.
dates, dried	59	63	1.1	0.9	67	71	4 oz.
figs, dried	124	76	0.6	1.6	140	86	4 oz.
grapefruit	18	18	1.0	1.0	40	40	8 oz.
grapes, green, seedless	8	13	1.6	0.6	18	29	8 oz.
lemons	17	11	0.6	1.6	20	12	4 oz.
olives, canned	106	17	0.2	6.2	120	19	4 oz.
orange	41	20	0.5	2.1	93	45	8 oz.
papaya	35	104	3.0	0.3	80	235	8 oz.
peach	9	19	2.2	0.5	20	44	8 oz.
pears, canned	5	7	1.4	0.7	6	8	4 oz.
pears, uncooked	8	11	1.3	0.8	19	25	8 oz.
pineapple	17	8	0.5	2.2	39	18	8 oz.
strawberries	21	21	1.0	1.0	24	24	4 oz.
tangerines	30	13	0.4	2.2	67	30	8 oz.
watermelon	7	10	1.4	0.7	16	23	8 oz.

MEATS	mg per 100 grams		P/Ca	Ca/P	mg per serving		serving
	calcium	phosph.	(bad)	(good)	calcium	phosph.	size
bacon, broiled or fried	14	224	16.1	0.1	16	254	4 oz.
bacon, Canadian	19	218	11.5	0.1	22	247	4 oz.
beef, pot roast or chuck roast	11	140	12.7	0.1	25	317	8 oz.
bologna	7	128	18.2	0.1	16	291	8 oz.
chicken chow mein	23	117	5.1	0.2	52	265	8 oz.
chicken liver, cooked	11	159	14.4	0.1	25	360	8 oz.
chicken, broiled	9	201	22.2	0.0	21	457	8 oz.
chicken, roast	11	265	24.0	0.0	25	602	8 oz.
chicken, fried	13	272	20.5	0.0	30	616	8 oz.
corned beef	9	93	10.3	0.1	21	211	8 oz.
frankfurter	5	102	20.1	0.0	12	231	8 oz.
hamburger	22	141	6.3	0.2	51	320	8 oz.
ham, cured, roast	9	172	19.5	0.1	20	390	8 oz.
lamb chops, broiled	9	156	17.7	0.1	20	354	8 oz.
pork chops, roast	10	232	23.4	0.0	23	526	8 oz.
steak, T-bone, porterhouse, rib	10	186	18.7	0.1	23	422	8 oz.
turkey, roast	11	300	27.2	0.0	25	680	8 oz.
TV dinner, meat loaf	19	117	6.1	0.2	43	265	8 oz.
TV dinner, turkey	37	124	3.4	0.3	84	281	8 oz.
veal cutlet, broiled	11	225	20.4	0.0	25	510	8 oz.

FISH AND SEAFOOD	mg per 100 grams		P/Ca	Ca/P	mg per serving		serving
	calcium	phosph.	(bad)	(good)	calcium	phosph.	size
crabmeat, canned	43	174	4.1	0.2	97	395	8 oz.
flounder, baked	23	349	14.9	0.1	53	792	8 oz.
halibut, broiled	16	252	15.4	0.1	37	571	8 oz.
kelp	1093	240	0.2	4.6	310	68	1 oz.
salmon, sockeye, canned	258	342	1.3	0.8	585	776	8 oz.
sardines, canned in oil	272	432	1.6	0.6	618	980	8 oz.
shrimp, cooked	72	190	2.6	0.4	163	431	8 oz.
tuna, canned in oil, drained	8	233	29.3	0.0	18	528	8 oz.

EGGS AND DAIRY PRODUCTS	mg per 100 grams		P/Ca	Ca/P	mg per serving		serving
	calcium	phosph.	(bad)	(good)	calcium	phosph.	size
cheese, American or cheddar	753	476	0.6	1.6	1708	1081	8 oz.
cheese, creamed cottage	94	152	1.6	0.6	214	345	8 oz.
cheese, parmesan	1143	782	0.7	1.5	1296	887	4 oz.
egg, raw, boiled, or poached	54	206	3.8	0.3	31	117	2 oz.
milk, human	33	13	0.4	2.5	76	30	8 oz.
skim milk	121	95	0.8	1.3	275	216	8 oz.
whole milk	118	93	0.8	1.3	267	210	8 oz.
yogurt, low-fat	120	94	0.8	1.3	272	213	8 oz.

SOUP	mg per 100 grams		P/Ca	Ca/P	mg per serving		serving
	calcium	phosph.	(bad)	(good)	calcium	phosph.	size
chicken noodle soup	4	15	3.8	0.3	9	34	8 oz.
ministrone	15	24	1.6	0.6	34	54	8 oz.
split pea soup	12	61	5.1	0.2	27	139	8 oz.

SAUCES AND CONDIMENTS	mg per 100 grams		P/Ca	Ca/P	mg per serving		serving
	calcium	phosph.	(bad)	(good)	calcium	phosph.	size
blackstrap molasses	685	85	0.1	8.1	194	24	1 oz.
French salad dressing	11	14	1.3	0.8	3	4	1 oz.
Italian salad dressing	10	4	0.4	2.5	3	1	1 oz.
kelp	1093	240	0.2	4.6	310	68	1 oz.
light molasses	165	45	0.3	3.7	47	13	1 oz.
maple syrup	105	8	0.1	13.1	30	2	1 oz.
mustard	124	134	1.1	0.9	35	38	1 oz.
soy sauce	82	104	1.3	0.8	23	29	1 oz.
tomato catsup	22	50	2.3	0.4	6	14	1 oz.

JUICES	mg per 100 grams		P/Ca	Ca/P	mg per serving		serving
	calcium	phosph.	(bad)	(good)	calcium	phosph.	size
apple juice	6	9	1.5	0.7	14	21	8 oz.
grapefruit juice	8	14	1.8	0.6	18	32	8 oz.
lemon juice	7	13	2.0	0.5	2	4	1 oz.
orange juice, fresh	11	17	1.5	0.7	25	39	8 oz.
orange juice, frozen concentrate	32	54	1.7	0.6	73	122	8 oz.
tomato juice	7	18	2.6	0.4	16	41	8 oz.

NUTS, SEEDS, AND NUT BUTTER	mg per 100 grams		P/Ca	Ca/P	mg per serving		serving
	calcium	phosph.	(bad)	(good)	calcium	phosph.	size
almonds, roasted and salted	234	504	2.2	0.5	266	572	4 oz.
cashews, unsalted	39	373	9.6	0.1	44	423	4 oz.
peanut butter	57	380	6.6	0.2	65	431	4 oz.
peanuts, roasted, salted	75	401	5.4	0.2	85	455	4 oz.
sesame seeds, whole	1160	616	0.5	1.9	1315	699	4 oz.
sesame seeds, hulled	110	592	5.4	0.2	125	671	4 oz.
sunflower seeds	120	837	7.0	0.1	136	949	4 oz.
walnuts	0	570		0.0	0	646	4 oz.

FRUITS	silicon
	mg per 100 grams
acerolas	7
apples	64
apricots	53
avocado	11
bananas	20
blackberries	51
blueberries	0
boysenberries	0
canteloupe	88
casaba	0
honeydew	0
muskmelon	88
cheries	66
coconut	88
cranberries	2
currants, black	20
dates	2
figs	35
lemons	4
limes	4
olives	7
oranges	4
papaya	4
peaches	2
pears	7
persimmons	0
plums	18
prunes	13
pomegranate	2
pumpkin	17
rasberries, black	18
rhubarb	2
strawberries	22
tangeriens	1
tomatoes	11
watermelon	11

VEGETABLES	silicon
	mg per 100 grams
alfalfa	0
artichokes	2
asperagus	2
beans, kidney	2
beans, lima	4
beans, string	2
beets	88
broccoli	22
brussels sprouts	2
cabbage	9
cabbage, savoy	104
carrots	22
cauliflower	33
celery	31
chard	7
corn	18
cucumbers	35
dandelion greens	135
eggplant	4
garlic	22
horseradish	225
kale	2
leeks	97
lettuce	86
lettuce, romaine	40
onions	99
parsley	38
parsnips	168
peas	2
bell peppers	33
potatoes, white	22
potatoes, sweet	20
radish	9
spinach	181
turnips	11

boron		
parts per million		
	lowest of several tests	highest of several tests
snap beans	10	73
cabbage	7	42
lettuce	6	37
tomatoes	5	36
spinach	12	88

REFERENCES
Chapter 1

1 Richards B. *Blood of the Moon*. ODAE Productions, Toronto, Ontario, 1992.

2 Utian, WH. Case Western Reserve Med School, Cleveland,OH.

3 Choay P; Lafond JL; Favier A. [Value of micronutrient supplements in the prevention or correction of disorders of menopause]. *Revue Francaise de Gynecologie et D Obstetrique* 1990; 85(12):702-5.

4 Metka M. [Osteoporosis & estrogens]. *Wiener Med Wochenschrift* 1990 Oct 15; 140(18-19):485-6.

5 Arnaud CD; Sanchez SD. The role of calcium in osteoporosis. *Annual Rev of Nutr* 1990; 10:397.

6 Cooper C; Barker, DJP. Risk Factors for Hip Fracture. *NEJM* 1995; 332(12):814-815.

7 Schneider HP; Doren M. [Treatment of osteoporosis]. *Zentralblatt fur Gynakologie* 1994; 116(12):691.

8 Doren M; Schneider HP. Identification & treatment of postmenopausal women at risk for development of osteoporosis. *Intl of Clin Pharmacology, Therapy, & Toxicology* 1992 Nov; (11):431-3.

9 Lee, JR. *Optimal Health Guidelines*, 1991.

10 Editorial, *Lancet* 1993; 341:151-2.

11 Ibid.

12 Hunt, RM. Book Review, *Infections in Bones & Joints*, *NEJM*; 332:615.

Chapter 2

1 Sher A; Rahman A. Role of diet on the enterohepatic recycling of estrogen in women taking contraceptive pills. *J of Pakistan Med Assoc* 1994 Sep; 44(9):213-5.

2 Ho KK; et al. Impact of short-term estrogen administration on GH. *J of Bone &Min Res* 1992; 7:8217.

3 Kroon UB, Silfverstolpe G, Tengborn L. The effects of transdermal estradiol & oral conjugated estrogens on haemostasis variables. *Thrombosis Haemostasis* 1994 Apr; 71(4):420-3

4 Balfour JA; Heel RC. Transdermal estradiol. A Rev. *Drugs* 1990; 40:561-82.

5 Di Carlo F. [Action of drugs in relation to the administration route]. *Min Endoc* 1989 Jan-Mar; 14(1):41.

6 Op cit, Balfour.

7 Op cit, Di Carlo.

8 Goretzlehner G. [Efficacy of different estrogens]. *Zentralblatt fur Gynakologie* 1989; 111:1093-100.

9 Ibid.

10 Vorster HH et al. Egg intake does not change. *Amer J of Clin Nutr* 1992 Feb; 55(2):400-10.

11 Schnohr P; et al. Egg consumption & HDL cholesterol. *J of Int Med* 1994 Mar; 235(3):249-51.

Chapter 3

1 *The Incredible Machine*, National Geographic Society, 1986, p 239.

2 Baird DT; Glasier AF. Drug therapy: hormonal contraception. *NEJM* 1993; 328:1543.

3 Kamen, B; *Everything You Wanted to Know About Potassium* (Novato, CA: Nutr Encounter, 1992).

4 Vasuvattakul S; et al. Kaliuretic response to aldosterone: influence of the content of potassium in the diet. *Amer J of Kidney Dis* 1993 Feb; 21(2):152-60.

5 Rhofes, R; Pflanzer, R. *Hum Phys* (Fort Worth, TX: Saunders , Harcourt Brace, 1992), p 435.

6 Ibid, p 1015.

7 Richard Kunin, MD, Personal communication, February 1, 1993.

8 Edgren RA. Clinical use of sex steroids, Year Book Med Publishers, Inc., 1980.

9 Godsand IF; Crook D. Update on metabolic effects of steroidal contraceptives & their relationship to cardiovascular disease risk. *Amer J of Ob & Gyn* 1994; 170:1528-36.

10 Ibid.

11 Op cit, Lee.

12 Ibid.

13 Darj E et al. Liver met during treatment with estradiol & natural prog. *Gyn End* 1993 Jun; 7(2):111.

Chapter 4

1 Posting on the WELL, electronic communication, 1993. <Athena>.

2 Richards B; *Blood of the Moon*. ODAE Productions, Toronto, Ontario, 1992.

3 Seligmann J; Gelman D. Is it sadness or madness? *Newsweek*, March 15, 1993, p 66.

4 Rhofes, R; Pflanzer, R. *Hum Physi* (Fort Worth, Texas: Saunders, Harcourt Brace, 1992), p 992.

5 Op cit, Kamen, Potassium.

6 Rosseel M; Schoors, D. Chewing gum & hypokalemia. *Lancet* 1993; 341:175.

7 Lane JD et al. Menstrual cycle effects on caffeine. *Eur J of Clin Pharmacology*, 1992; 43(5):543-6.

8 Shephard, BD; Shephard, CA. *Complete Guide to Women's Health* (NY: Penguin books, 1990), p 443.

9 Lever J; Brush MG. *Premenstrual Tension* (New York: McGraw Hill, 1981), p 146.

10 Seaman, B; Seamn G. *Women & the Crisis in Sex Hormones* (NY: Rawson Associates, 1977), p 142.

11 Stewart F; et al. *My Body, My Health* (New York: John Wiley & Sons, 1979), p 387.

12 Salvat J; Jolles C. [Progesterone, progestagens in premenstrual syndrome, the perimenopause and the menopause]. *Schweizerische Rundschau fur Medizin Praxis* 1995 Jan 17; 84(3):70.

13 Facchinetti F; et al. Changes of opioid modulation of the hypothalamo-pituitary-adrenal axis in patients with severe PMS. *Psychosomatic Med* 1994 Sep-Oct; 56(5):418-22.

14 Menkes DB; Coates DC; Fawcett JP. Acute tryptophan depletion aggravates premenstrual syndrome. *J of Affective Disorders*, 1994 Sep; 32(1):37-44.

15 Facchinetti F; et al. Neuroendocrine changes in luteal function in patients with PMS. *J of Clin End & Met* 1993 May; 76(5):1123-7.

16 Chuong CJ. Periovulatory beta-endorphin levels in PMS. *Ob & Gyn* 1994 May; 83(5 Pt 1):755-60.

17 Chuong CJ et al. Zinc & copper levels in PMS. *Fertility & Sterility*, 1994 Aug; 62(2):313-20.

18 Piccoli A; et al. Reduction in urinary prostaglandin excretion in PMS. *J of Rep Med* 1993; 38:941.

19 Posaci C; et al.. Plasma copper, zinc & mg levels in PMS. *Acta Ob et Gyn Scan* 1994 Jul; 73:452.

20 Kuczmierczyk AR; Labrum AH; Johnson CC.The relationship between mood, somatization, & alexithymia inpremenstrual syndrome. *Psychosomatics* 1995 Jan-Feb; 36(1):26-32.

21 Op cit, Facchinetti F et al.

22 Mansfield MJ; et al. Anorexia nervosa, athletes, & amenorrhea. *Ped Clin of N Am* 1989 Jun; 36:533.

23 Fong AKH; Kretsch MJ. Changes in dietary intake, urinary nitrogen, & urinary volume across the menstrual cycle. *Amer J of Clin Nutr* 1993; 57:43-6.

24 Rossignol AM; Bonnlander H. Prevalence & severity of the premenstrual syndrome. Effects of foods & beverages that are sweet or high in sugar content. *J of Reproductive Med* 1991 Feb; 3:131-6.

25 Rabin DS; et al. Hypothalamic-pituitary-adrenal function/PMS. *J of Clin End & Met* 1990; 71-1158.

26 Steinberg S; et al.. Tryptophan in the treatment of late luteal phase dysphoric disorder: a pilot study. *J of Psychiatry & Neuroscience* 1994 Mar; 19(2):114-9.

27 Hesla JS; et al. Superoxide dismutase activity. *J of Repr & Ferty* 1992 Aug; 95(3):915-24.

28 Caufriez A. Menstrual disorders in adolescence. *Hormone Res* 1991; 36(3-4):156.

Chapter 5

1 Burckhardt P; Michel C. The peak bone mass concept. *Clin Rheumatology* 1989 Jun; 8 Suppl 2:16.

2 Metzger DA; Hammond CB. Are estrogens indicated for the treatment of postmenopausal women? *Drug Intel & Clin Pharm* 1988 Jun; 22(6):493-6.

3 Ellis JM et al. A deficiency of vitamin B6 is a plausible molecular basis of the retinopathy of patients with diabetes mellitus. *Biophysical Res Communications* 1991 Aug 30; 179(1):615-9.

4 Bernstein AL. Vitamin B6 in clin neurology. *Ann of NY Academy of Science* 1990; 585:250-60.

5 Pascual E; et al. Higher incidence of CTS in oophorectomized women. *Brit J Rheum* 1991; 30(1):60.

6 Zamboni M; et al. Body fat distribution in pre- & post-menopausal women: metabolic & anthropometric variables & their inter-relationships. *International J of Obesity* 1992 Jul; 16(7):495-504.

7 Matthews KA; et al. Influences of natural menopause on psychological characteristics & symptoms of middle-aged healthy women. *J of Consulting & Clin Psychology* 1990 Jun; 58(3):345-51.

8 van Beresteyn EC; et al. Contributions of ovarian failure & aging to blood pressure in normotensive perimenopausal women: a mixed longitudinal study. *Amer J of Epid* 1989 May; 129(5):947-55.

9 Hafner H et al. Oestradiol enhances vulnerability threshold for schizophrenia . Evidence from an epidemiological study & animal exps. *Eur Arch of Psychy & Clin Neuroscience* 1991; 241(1):65-8.

10 Op cit, Metzger & Hammond.

11 Fugere P. [Replacement hormone therapy: the earlier the menopause, the greater the importance of treatment (interview)]. *Union Mede du Canada* 1992 Mar-Apr; 121(2):125-9.

12 Kin K et al. Bone mineral density of the spine in normal Japanese subjects using dual-energy X-ray absorptiometry: effect of obesity & menopausal status. *Calcified Tissue Int* 1991 Aug; 49:101.

13 Beard MK. Atrophic vaginitis. Can it be prevented? *Postgraduate Med* 1992 May; 91:257.

14 Zaridze D; et al. Diet, alcohol consumption & reproductive factors in a case-control study of breast cancer in Moscow. *International J of Cancer* 1991 Jun 19; 48(4):493-501.

15 Cummings SR; et al. Bone density at various sites for prediction of hip fractures. *Lancet* 1993; 341:72.

16 Prior JC; Vigna YM; Alojado N. Progesterone & the prevention of osteoporosis. *Canadian J of Obstetrics & Gynecology & Women's Health Care* 1991; 3:178-84.

17 Leidy LE. Early age at menopause among left-handed women. *Ob & Gyn* 1990; 76(6):1111-4.

18 Tajtakova M; et al. [The effect of smoking on menopause *J of Obesity* 1992 Jul; 16(7):495-504.

19 Key TJ; et al. Cigarette smoking & steroid hormones in women. *J of Steroid Biochemistry & Molecular Biology* 1991 Oct; 39(4A):529-34.

20 Adlercreutz H et al. Dietary phyto-estrogens & the menopause in Japan. *Lancet* 1992; 339:1233.

21 Barnard RM; et al. Effect of fever on menopausal hot flashes. *Maturitas* 1992 Mar; 14(3):181-8.

22 Shaver J; et al. Sleep patterns & stability in perimenopausal women. *Sleep* 1988 Dec; 11(6):556-61.

23 Kronenberg F. Hot flashes: epidemiology & physiology. *Annals of the New York Academy of Sciences* 1990; 592:52-86; discussion 123-33.

24 *Obstetrics & Gynecology* 1994.

25 Roberts PJ. The menopause & hormone replacement therapy: views of women in general practice receiving hormone replacement therapy. *British J of General Practice* 1991 Oct; 41(351):421-4.

26 Aina AO. Investigation into Nigerians. *J of the Med Assoc of Thailand* 1992; 75:168.

27 Zamboni M et al. Body fat distribution in pre- & post-menopausal women: metabolic & anthropometric variables & their inter-relationships. *Int J of Obesity* 1992 Jul; 16(7):495-504.

28 Roberts PJ. The menopause & hormone replacement therapy: views of women in general practice receiving hormone replacement therapy. *British J of General Practice* 1991 Oct; 41(351):421-4.

Chapter 6

1 Kelly PJ; et al. Interaction of genetic & environmental influences. *Osteo Int* 1990 Oct; 1:56-60.

2 Hirota T; et al. Effect of diet & lifestyle on bone mass in Asian young women. *AJCN* 1992; 55:1168.

3 Tylavsky FA; et al. Familial resemblance of radial bone mass between premenopausal mothers & their college-age daughters. *Calcified Tissue International* 1989 Nov; 45(5):265-72.

4 Pollitzer WS; Anderson JJ. Ethnic & genetic differences in bone mass: a rev with a hereditary vs environmental perspective [published erratum appears in Amer J of Clin Nutr, 1990 Jul; 52(1):181]. *Amer J of Clin Nutr* 1989 Dec; 50(6):1244-59.

5 Rhofes, R; Pflanzer, R. *Human Physiology* (Fort Worth, TX: Saunders, Harcourt Brace, 1992), p 915.

6 Burton, BT. *Human Nutr* (New York: McGraw-Hill, 1976), p 129.

7 Nordin BEC; et al. Calcium & bone met in old age. *Nutr in Old Age*, ed Carlson LA (Uppsala, Sweden: Swedish Nutr Foundation, 1972).

8 Albanese AA. *Current Topics in Nutr & Disease*, vol 3: *Nutr for the Elderly* (NY: Alan R Liss), Lutwak L. Continuing need for dietary calcium through life. *Geriatrics* 1974; 29:171.

9 Macy IG. *Nutr & Chemical Growth in Childhood* (Springfield, IL: Charles C Thomas, 1942).

10 Lees B; et al. Differences in proximal femur bone density over two centuries. *Lancet* 1993; 341:673.

11 Cummings SR; et al. Risk factors for hip fracture in white women. *NEJM* 1995; 767-773.

12 Cummings SR; et al. Bone density at various sites for prediction of hip fractures. *Lancet* 1993; 341.

13 Hernandez-Avila M; et al. Caffeine & other predictors of bone density. *Epidemiology* 1993;4:128.

14 Burckhardt P; Michel C. The peak bone mass concept. *Clin Rheumatology*, 1989 Jun 8; S2:16-21.

15 Kelly PJ; Eisman JA; Sambrook PN. Interaction of genetic & environmental influences on peak bone density. *Osteoporosis International* 1990 Oct; 1(1):56-60.

16 Kritz-Silverstein D; et al. Pregnancy & lactation as determinants. *Amer J of Epid* 1992 Nov; 136:1052.

17 Op cit, Lutwak.

18 Op cit, Cummings, *NEJM*.

19 Kamen B. *Startling New Facts About Osteoporosis* (Novato, California: Nutr Encounter, 1992).

20 Nilsson BE; et al. Changes in bone mass in alcoholics. *Clin Ortho & Related Res* 1973; 90:229.

21 Meghji S. Bone remodelling. *British Dental J* 1992 Mar 21; 172(6):235-42.

22 Ericson JE; Smith DR; Flegal AR. Skeletal concentrations of lead, cadmium, zinc, & silver in ancient North Amer Pecos Indians. *Environmental Health Perspectives* 1991 Jun; 93:217-23.

23 Saltzman BE; et al. Total body burdens & tissue concentrations of lead, cadmium, copper, zinc, & ash in 55 human cadavers. *Environmental Res* 1990 Aug; 52(2):126-45.

24 Lee JR. *Optimal Health Guidelines*, 1991.

25 Op cit, Cummings, *NEJM*.

Chapter 7

1 Lee, JR. Hormonal & nutritional aspects of osteoporosis. *Health & Nutr* 1991; 6:4.

2 Slootweg MC; et al. Oestrogen & progestogen synergistically stimulate human & rat osteoblast proliferation. *J of End* 1992 May; 133(2):R5-8.

3 Tremollieres F; Pouilles JM; Ribot C. [Postmenopausal bone loss. Role of progesterone & androgens]. *Presse Mede* 1992 Jun 6; 21(21):989-93.

4 Hedlund LR et al. Effect of age & menopause on bone. *J of Bone & Mineral Res* 1989; 4(4):639-42.

5 Amano K et al. [Effect of suppletory estrogen or 1,25(OH)D3 on bone mineral content]. Nippon Sanka Fujinka Gakkai Zasshi. *Acta Obstetrica et Gynaecologica Japonica* 1992 Jul; 44(7):833-6.

6 Op cit, Hedlund & Gallagher.

7 National Inst of Health, Consnesus Conf: Osteoporosis. *J of the Amer Med Assoc* 1984; 252:799.

8 Op cit, Lee, *Health & Nutr*, p 4.

9 Booher DL. Estrogen supplements in menopause. *Cleveland Clin J of Med* 1990 Mar-Apr; 57(2):15.

10 Cummings SR et al. Bone density at various sites for prediction of hip fractures. *Lancet* 1993; 341:72.

11 Love RR et al. Effects of tamoxifen on women with breast cancer. *NEJM* 1992; 326:852-6.

12 Cooper C; Barker, DJP. Risk factors for hip fracture. *NEJM* 1995; 332:814-815.

13 Chrischilles E et al. Costs and health effects of osteoporotic fractures. *Bone* 1994; 15:377-73.

14 *Osteoporosis International* (8).

15 John Lee, personal communication, March, 1993.

16 Metka M. [Osteoporosis & estrogens]. *Wiener Medizinische Wochenschrift* 1990 Oct 15; 140:485-6.

17 Lutwak L. Continuing need for dietary calcium through life. *Geriatrics* 1974; 29:171.

Chapter 8

1 Electronic mail on The Well with Professor William H Calvin, University of Washington, January, 1993.

2 Forbes AP. Fuller Albright. His concept of postmenopausal osteoporosis & what came of it. *Clin Orthopaedics & Related Res* 1991 Aug; (269):128-41.

3 National Institute of Health, Consnesus Conference: Osteoporosis. *JAMA* 1984; 252:799.

4 Lee, L. Estrogen, Progesterone & Female Problems. *Earthletter* 1991 June; 1(2):1.

5 Reinisch JM; et al. Effects of prenatal exposure to (DES). *Hormones & Behavior* 1992 Mar; 26(1):62-75.

6 Reinisch JM; et al. Hormonal contributions. *PsychoneuroEnd* 1991; 16(1-3):213-78.

7 Telang NT; et al. Induction by estrogen metabolite. *J of the National Cancer Institute* 1992 Apr; 84:634.

8 Schlehofer B; Blettner M; Wahrendorf J. Assoc between brain tumors & menopausal status. *J of the National Cancer Institute* 1992 Sep 2; 84(17):1346-9.

9 Burgat V. [Residues of drugs of vet use in food]. *Revue du Praticien* 1991 Apr 11; 41(11):985-90.

10 Witkamp RF; Korstanje C; van Miert AS. [Toxicological & pharmacological effects of the use of bovine somatotropin in dairy farming]. *Tijdschrift voor Diergeneeskunde* 1990 Sep 1; 115(17):780-8.

11 Nagasawa H. Physiological significance of hormones & related substances in milk with special reference to prolactin: an overview. *Endocrine Regulations* 1991 Jun; 25(1-2):90-7.

12 Karg H. [The current status & risk evaluation of the use of hormone preparations in food producing animals]. *Monatsschrift Kinderheilkunde* 1990 Jan; 138(1):2-5.

13 Moishezon-Blank N. Commentary on the possible effect of hormones in food on human growth. *Med Hypotheses* 1992 Aug; 38(4):273-7.

14 Ibid.

15 Gambrell RD Jr. Use of progestogens. *Intnl J of Fertility* 1989 Sep-Oct; 34(5):315-21.

16 Markovitz JH et al. Psychological, biological & health behavior predictors of blood pressure changes in middle-aged women. *J of Hypertension* 1991 May; 9(5):399-406.

17 Op cit, Kamen, *Osteoporosis* .

18 Hermier D et al. Alterations in plasma lipoproteins & apolipoproteins associated with estrogen-induced hyperlipidemia in the laying hen. *European J of Biochemistry* 1989 Sep 1; 184(1):109-18.

19 Wells, RG. "Should All Postmenopausal Women Receive HRT?" *Senior Patient* 1989; 1:65

20 Manson JE. Postmenopausal HRT & atherosclerotic disease. *Amer Heart J* 1994; 128:1337-43.

21 Kamen, B. *New Facts About Fiber* (Novato, California: Nutr Encounter, 1991), p 47..

22 Whitehead MI et al. The role & use of progestogens. *Ob & Gyny* 1990 Apr; 75(4 Suppl):59S-76S.

23 Henderson BE; Bernstein L. The international variation in breast cancer rates: an epidemiological assessment. *Breast Cancer Res & Treatment* 1991 May; 18 Suppl 1:S11-7.

24 Kalkhoven E et al. Synthetic progestins induce breast tumor cell lines. *Mol & Cell Endocrin* 1994; 102:45.

25 White JO; et al. Human squamous cervical carcinoma cell line. *Intnl J of Cancer* 1992 Sep 9; 52(2):247.

26 Chen A; Huminer D. The role of estrogen receptors in the development of gallstones & gallbladder cancer. *Med Hypotheses* 1991 Nov; 36(3):259-60.

27 Adams JB. Enzymatic regulation of estradiol-17 beta concentrations in human breast cancer cells. *Breast Cancer Res & Treatment* 1992 Mar; 20(3):145-54.

28 Cantor KP et al. Bladder cancer, parity, & age at first birth. *Cancer Causes & Control*, 1992 Jan, 3(1):57.

29 Cagle PT; Mody DR; Schwartz MR. Estrogen & progesterone receptors in bronchogenic carcinoma. & colorectal cancer cell lines. *Cancer* 1989 Jun 1; 63(11):2148-51.

30 Andren-Sandberg A; et al. Influence of sex hormones on pancreatic cancer. *Int J of Panc* 1990; 7:167.

31 Harrison JD; Watson S; Morris DL. The effect of sex hormones and tamoxifen on the growth of human gastric and colorectal cancer cell lines. *Cancer* 1989 Jun 1; 63(11):2148-51.

32 Colin C. [Hormone substitution therapy in menopause & risk of breast cancer]. *Revue Francaise de Gynecologie et D Obstetrique* 1991 Jan; 86(1):27-8.

33 Reinisch JM; Sanders SA. Effects of prenatal exposure to (DES). *Hormones & Behavior* 1992 Mar; (1):62.

34 Castelo-Branco C; et al. Transvaginal sonography of the endometrium. *Maturitas* 1994; 19:59.

Chapter 9

1 Op cit, Lee, *Health & Nutr*, 6:4, winter 1991, p 4.

2 Prior, J.C; Vigna, Y.; Alojada, N. Progesterone & the prevention of osteoporosis. *Canadian J of Ob/Gyn & Women's Health Care* 1991; 3(4):181.

3 Prior, JC; Wark, JD; Barr, SI. The prevention & treatment of osteoporosis. *Lancet* 1993; 328:65-6.

4 Tremollieres F; et al. [Postmenopausal bone loss. *Presse Mede* 1992 Jun 6; 21(21):989-93.

5 Lee, J. Is Natural Progesterone the Missing Link in Osteoporosis Prevention & Treatment? *Med Hypotheses* 1991; 35:316-318.

6 Coen D; Terzian E; Magrini N. The prevention & treatment of osteoporosis. *Lancet* 1993; 328:65-6.

7 Gallagher JC; et al. Effects of therapy vary on different parts of the skelaton. *Clin Res* 1986; 34:927A.

8 Gallagher JC; et al. Comparison of estrogen & progestin therapy. *Int Nat Conf CT* 1986.

9 Prior, J.C. Progesterone as a one-trophic hormone. *Endocrine Revs* 1990; 11(2):394.

10 Peat, R. *Nutr for Women* (Centotech: Oswego, Oregon, 1981), p 25-26.

11 Hargrove, J; et al. Menopausal hormone replacement therapy with continuous daily oral micronized estradiol & progesterone. *Obstetrics & Gynecology* 1989 April; 73(4).

12 Personal interview with Martin Milner, N.D., January 14, 1993, Las Vegas.

13 Ibid.

14 Prior JC. Progesterone as a bone-trophic hormone. *Endocrine Revs* 1990 May; 11(2):386-98.

15 Wysowski DK; et al. Use of menopausal estrogens & medroxyprogesterone in the US. *Ob & Gyn* 1995; 85:6.

16 Barengolts EI; et al. Effects of progesterone on postovariectomy bone loss in aged rats. *J of Bone & Mineral Res* 1990 Nov; 5(11):1143-7.

17 Lindsay R. The effect of sex steroids on the skeleton in premenopausal women. *Amer J of Obstetrics & Gynecology* 1992 Jun; 166(6 Pt 2):1993-6.

18 Op cit, Prior.

19 Ibid.

20 Blaakaer J; et al. The pituitary-gonadal axis in women with benign or malignant ovarian tumors. *Acta Endocrinologica* 1992 Aug; 127(2):127-30.

Chapter 10

1 Eaton SB; Nelson DA. Calcium in evolutionary perspective. *Amer J of Clin Nutr* 1991; 54:Sl:281S-7S.

2 Heany, R.P. "Thinking straight about calcium." *NEJM*, 1993; 328:503-5.

3 Lees B; et al. Differences in proximal femur bone density over two centuries. *Lancet* 1993; 341:673:675.

4 Op cit, Heany.

5 Ettinger B. Role of calcium in preserving the skeletal health. *Southern Med J* 1992 Aug; 85(8):2S22-30.

6 Angus RM; et al. Dietary intake & bone mineral density. *Bone & Mineral* 1988 Jul; 4(3):265-77.

7 De Lucas, H. The Latest information on vitamin D & bone status. *Complimentary Med* 1986; 13.

8 Reginster JY et al. Treatment of osteoporosis: current data. *Revue du Rhumatisme* 1994; 61:155S.

9 *British Med J* 1984; 289:1103.

10 Chalmers, J. Geographical Variations in Senile Osteoporosis. *J of Bone & Joint Surgery* 1970; 52B:667.

11 Charles P. Calcium absorption & calcium bioavailability. *J of Int Med* 1992 Feb; 231(2):161-8.

12 Koshiyama; et al. Vitamin-D-receptor-gene polymorphism & bone loss. *Lancet* 1995; 345:990-91.

13 Cooper C; Barker DJP. Risk factors for hip fracture. *NEJM* 1995; 332:814-815.

14 Strain JJ. A reassessment of diet & osteoporosis—role for copper. *Med Hypothesis* 1988; 27(4):333-8.

15 Reid IR; et al. Effect of calcium supplementation on bone loss. *NEJM* 1993; 328:460-4.

16 Cummings SR; et al. Bone density at various sites for prediction of hip fractures. *Lancet* 1993; 341:72.

17 Cummings SR; et al. Risk factors for hip fracture in white women. *NEJM* 1995; 328:767-773.

18 Arnaud CD; Sanchez SD. The role of calcium in osteoporosis. *Ann Rev of Nutr* 1990; 10:397-414.

19 Fujita T et al. Comparison of osteo & ca bt Japan & US. *Proc of Soc Exper Bio & Med* 1992 ; 200:149.52.

20 Riis, B; Thomsen, K; Christiannsen, C. Does Calcium Supplementation Prevent Postmenopausal Bone Loss? *NEJM* 1987; 316:173.

21 Sheikh, MS; et al. Gastrointestinal absorption of ca from milk & ca salts," *NEJM* 1987; 317:532.

22 Stevenson, JC. "Dietary Calcium & Hip Fracture," *Lancet* 1988; 2:1318.

23 Dudl, RJ et al, Evaluation of Intravenous Calcium Therapy for Osteoporosis, *Amer J of Med* 1973 55:631.

24 Strier KB. Menu for a monkey. *Natural History* 1993; 102:34-42.

Chapter 11

1 Recker, RR. The effect of milk supplements on calcium metabolism.. AJCN 1968; 41:254.

2 Sheehy, G. *The Silent Passage*, (New York, Random House, 1992) p 103.

3 *J of Clin Pediatric Dentistry* 1991; 16:38.

4 *Roczniki Panstwowego Zakladu Higieny* 1989; 40:266.

5 Lee, J.R. Hormonal & nutritional aspects of osteoporosis. *Health & Nutr* 1991; 6:7.

6 Riggs BL; et al. Effect of flouride treatment on fracture rate. *NEJM* 1990; 322:802-9.

7 Sowers, FR; et al. A prospective study of bone mineral content & fracture in communities with differential fluoride exposure. *Amer J of Epidemiology* 1991; 133:649-660.

8 Jacobsen, SJ; et al. Regional variation in incidence of hip fracture. *JAMA* 1990; 264:500-502.

9 Cooper C; et al. Water flouridation & hip fracture. *J of the Amer Med Assoc* 1991; 266:513.

10 Danielson C. *J of the Amer Med Assoc* 1992 August 12.

11 Randal J. USA: Another flap over fluoride. *Lancet* 1990; 335:282.

12 Revis. Chlorinated water & reduced ca; hypercholesterolemic effect. *Clin Res* 1983; 31:865.

13 Report issued by North Marin Water District, Novato, California, 1991.

14 Arnaud CD; Sanchez SD. The role of calcium in osteoporosis. *Ann Rev of Nutr* 1990; 10:397-414.

15 Rader JI. Anti-nutritive effects of dietary tin. *Advances in Exp Med & Biology* 1991; 289:509-24.

16 Alfrey A. Aluminum intoxication. *NEJM* 1983.

17 Kiiskinen A; et al. Effect of prolonged physical training on the development of connective tissues. In *Metabolic Adaptation to Prolonged Physical Exercise* (Basel: Birkhauser Verlag, 1975), pp 253-61.

18 Steinhaus AH. Chronic effects of exercise. *Physiological Revs* 1933; 13:103-47.

19 Cummings SR et al. Risk factors for hip fracture in white women. *NEJM* 1995; 328:767-773.

20 Caffeine causes loss of calcium from bone. *Calcified Tissue International* 1992 Dec; 51(6):424-8.

21 Hunt IF; et al. Food & nutrient intake of Seventh-day Adventist. *Amer J of Clin Nutr* 1988; 48:S:850-1.

22 Op cit, Cummings.

23 Marsh AG; et al. Vegetarian lifestyle & bone mineral density. *Amer J of Clin Nutr* 1988; 48:837.

24 Pouilles JM; Tremollieres F; Ribot C. [Comparative effects of sodium fluoride & hormonal replacement therapy on bone. *Revue du Rhumatisme et des Maladies Osteo-Articulaires* 1992 Feb; 59(2):103-13.

25 Haddock DA. A simple way to manage menopause. *Postgraduate Med* 1990 Sep 1; 88(3):131-5, 138.

26 Burckhardt P; Michel C. The peak bone mass concept. *Clin Rheumatology* 1989; 8 Suppl 2:16-21.

27 Kelly PJ; Eisman JA; Sambrook PN. Interaction of genetic & environmental influences on peak bone density. *Osteoporosis International* 1990 Oct; 1(1):56-60.

28 Seelig MS. The requirement of magnesium by the normal adult. *AJCN* 1964, 14:342-90.

29 Prior JC; Vigna YM; McKay DW. Reproduction for the athletic woman. New understandings of physiology & management. *Sports Med* 1992 Sep; 14(3):190-9.

30 Strain JJ. A reassessment of diet & osteo;role for copper. *Med Hypotheses* 1988; 27(4):333-8.

31 Prince RL; et al. Prevention of postmenopausal osteoporosis. A comparative study of exercise, calcium

32 Op cit, Cummings.

Chapter 12

1 Personal interviews with Robert Cathcart, M.D 1990-93, San Francisco.

2 Nordin BE; Morris HA. Osteoporosis & vitamin D. *J of Cellular Biochemistry* 1992 May; 49(1):19-25.

3 Lee, J.R. Hormonal & Nutral Aspects of Osteoporosis. *Health & Nutr* 1991; 6:7.

4 Johnson K; et al. Preventive nutr: disease-spec/dietary interventions. *Geriatrics* 1992; 47(11):39-40, 45.

5 Op cit, Lee.

6 Kamen B. *Osteoporosis: What It Is, How to Prevent It, How to Stop It* (New York: Pinnacle, 1984), p 102.

7 Kunin RA. *Mega-Nutr for Women* (New York: McGraw-Hill, 1983), p 159.

8 Gogu SR; et al. Protection of zidovudine-induced toxicity against murine erythroid progenitor cells by vitamin E. *Experimental Hematology* 1991 Aug; 19(7):649-52.

9 Kaufmann K. *Silica: The Forgotten Nutrient* (British Colombia, Canada: Alive Books, 1990).

10 Pennington JA. Silicon in foods & diets. *Food Additives & Contaminants* 1991 Jan-Feb; 8(1):97-118.

11 Villareal CP; Juliano BO. Variability in contents of thiamine & riboflavin in brown rice, crude oil in brown rice & bran-polish, & silicon in hull of IR rices. *Plant Foods for Human Nutr* 1989; 39:287.

·12 Nielsen, FH; et al. Boron enhances & mimics some effects of estrogen therapy in postmenopausal women. *J of Trace Elements & Experimental Med* 1992; 5:237-46.

13 Hunt CD; Shuler TR; Mullen LM. Concentration of boron & other elements in human foods & personal-care products. *J of the Amer Dietetic Assoc* 1991 May; 91(5):558-68.

14 Mann J; Inman W. Oral contraceptives & death from myocardial infarction. *British Med J* 1975; 2:841.

15 Kamen B. *The Chromium Diet, Supplement & Exercise Strategy* (Novato, CA: Nutr Encounter, 1990).

16 Raisz LG; Kream BE. Regulation of bone formation. Part 2. *NEJM* 1983; 309:83-9.

17 *Cancer Letters* 1992 Oct 21; 66(3):207-16.

18 *Carcinogenesis*, 1992 Oct; 13(10):1847-51.

19 Babal K. *Nutr & Meganutrients* (Los Angeles, 1993).

20 Personal interview, Martin Milner, N.D., Las Vegas, 1993.

21 Phipps WR; et al. Effect of flax seed ingestion on the menstrual cyble. *J Clin Endocrinol Metab* 1993; 77:1215.

22 Choay P; Lafond JL; Favier A. [Value of micronutrient supplements in the prevention or correction of disorders accompanying menopause]. *Rev Francaise de Gyn et D Obstetrique* 1990 Dec; 85(12):702.

23 Benova DK. Anticlastogenic effects of a polyvitamin product, 'Pharmavit', on gamma-ray induction of somatic & germ cell chromosome aberrations in the mouse. *Mut Res* 1992 Oct; 269(2):251-8.

24 Franceschi RT. The role of ascorbic acid in mesenchymal differentiation. *Nutr Revs* 1992; 50:65.

25 Khan PK; Sinha SP. Antimutagenic efficacy of higher doses of vitamin C. *Mut Res* 1993 Jan; 298:157.

26 Lupulescu A. Ultrastructure & cell surface studies of cancer cells following vitamin C administration. *Experimental & Toxicologic Pathology* 1992 Mar; 44(1):3-9.

27 Ghosh A; et al. Relative protection given by extract of Phyllanthus emblica fruit & anequivalent amount of vitamin C against caesium chloride. *Food & Chemical Toxicology* 1992 Oct; 30(10):865-9.

28 Posaci C; et al. Plasma copper, zinc and mg levels in PMS. *Acta Obstet et Gyn Scand* 1994; 73:452-5.

29 Eisele PH; et al. Skeletal lesions & anemia associated with ascorbic acid deficiency in juvenile rhesus macaques. *Laboratory Animal Care* 1992 Jun; 42(3):245-9.

30 Arnaud CD; Sanchez SD. The role of calcium in osteoporosis. *Ann Rev of Nutr* 1990; 10:397-414.

31 Cruz ML; et al. Effect of chronic maternal dietary magnesium deficiency on placental calcium transport. *J of the Amer College of Nutr*; 1992 Feb; 11(1):87-92.

32 Rubinacci A; et al. [Influence of Nutr, age & vitamin D status on fasting urinary excretion of calcium in postmenopausal women]. *Minerva Medica* 1992 Oct; 83(10):601-8.

33 Khaw KT; Sneyd MJ; Compston J. Bone density parathyroid hormone & 25-hydroxyvitamin D concentrations in middle aged women. *British Med J* 1992 Aug 1; 305(6848):273-7.

34 Charles P. Calcium absorption & calcium bioavailability. *J of Int Med* 1992; 231(2):161-8.

35 Hamilton SJ; Buhl KJ. Acute toxicity of boron, molybdenum, & selenium to fry of chinook salmon & coho salmon. *Archives of Environmental Contamination & Toxicology* 1990; 19:366-73.

36 Nielsen FH; et al. Magnesium & methionine deprivation affectthe response of rats to boron deprivation. *Biological Trace Element Res* 1988; 17:91-107.

37 Nielsen, FH. New essential trace elements for the life sciences. *Bio Trace El Res* 1990; 26-27:599-611.

38 Nielsen FH. Ultratrace minerals mythical elixirs or nutrients of concern? Boletin - *Asociacion Medica de Puerto Rico* 1991 Mar; 83(3):131-3.

39 Newnham RE. Agricultural practices affect arthritis. *Nutr & Health* 1991; 7(2):89-100.

40 Leicht E; Biro G. Mechanisms of hypocalcaemia in the Clin form of severe magnesium deficit in the human. *Magnesium Res* 1992 Mar; 5(1):37-44.

41 Seelig MS. The requirement of magnesium by the normal adult. *Amer J of Clin Nutr* 1964; 14:342-90.

42 Mancinella A.[Silicon, a trace element essential for living organisms. Recent knowledge on its preventive role in atherosclerotic process, aging & neoplasms]. *Clinica Terapeutica* 1991 Jun 15; 137(5):343-50.

43 Carlisle EM. Silicon as a trace nutrient. *Science of the Total Environment* 1988 Jul 1; 73(1-2):95-106.

44 Reginster JY et al. Treatment of osteoporosis. *Rev du Rhumatisme* 1994; 61:155S.

Chapter 13

1 Khashaeva TKh; Magataeva MN; Tsadkina GG. [Clinico-immuno-hormonal parallels in obese women in the climacteric period]. *Akusherstvo i Ginekologiia* 1991 Jul; (7):59-63.

2 Schoutens A; et al. Serum triiodothyronine, bone turnover, & bone mass changes in euthyroid pre- & postmenopausal women. *Calcified Tissue International*, 1991 Aug; 49(2):95-100.

3 Koga M; Nakao H; Sato B. Effects of retinoic acid on estrogen- & thyroid hormone-induced growth in a newly established rat pituitary tumor cell line. *J of Steroid biochemistry & Molecular Biochemistry* 1992 Oct; 43:263.

4 Maruo T; et al. A role for thyroid hormone in the induction of ovulation & corpus luteum function. *Hormone Res* 1992; 37 Suppl 1:12-8.

5 Forsyth IA. The mammary gland. *Baillieres Clin End & Met* 1991 Dec; 5:809.

6 Matsuo H; et al. [Modification of endocrine function of trophoblasts by thyroid hormone]. Nippon Sanka Fujinka Gakkai Zasshi. *Acta Obstetrica et Gynaecologica Japonica* 1991 Nov; 43(11):1533-8.

7 Martinez, M; Derksen D; Kapsner P. Making sense of hypothyroidism. *Postgrad Med* 1993; 93(6):135.
8 Urban RJ. NeuroEnd of aging in the male & female. *End & Met Clinics of NA* 1992; 21(4):921.31.
9 Martinez, M et al. Making sense of hypothyroidism. *Postgraduate Med* 1993; 93(6):135.
10 Rosen CJ; Adler RA. Longitudinal changes in lumbar bone density among thyrotoxic patients after attainment of euthyroidism. *Jnl of Clin End & Met* 1992 Dec; 75(6):1531-4.
11 Coindre JM; et al. Bone loss in hypothyroidism with hormone replacement: a histomorphometric study. *Archives of Int Med* 1986; 146(1):48-53.
12 Stall GM; et al. Accelerated bone loss in hypothyroid patients overtreated with L-thyroxine. *Annals of Int Med* 1990; 113(4):265-9.
13 Franklyn JA; et al. Long-term thyroxine treatment & bone mineral density. *Lancet* 1992; 340:9-13.
14 Kronfol Z. Stress & immunity. *Lancet* 1993; 341:881-2.
15 Kovalenko AN; Sushko VA; Fedirko MI. [The hormonal functions regulating carbohydrate Met in participants in the cleanup of the sequelae of the accident at the Chernobyl Atomic Electric Power Station with a neurocirculatory dystonia syndrome]. *Vrachebnoe Delo* 1992 Jun; (6):52-5.
16 Kamen B. *Osteoporosis: What It Is, How to Prevent It, How to Stop It* (NY: Pinnacle, 1984). p 36.
17 Moyers B. *Healing and the Mind* (New York: Doubleday, 1993), p xi.
18 Verma S; et al. Superoxide dismutase activation in thyroid & suppression in adrenal. Novel pituitary regulatory routes. *Febs Letters* 1991 May 6; 282(2):310-2.
19 McMahon A; et al. Regulation of tyrosine hydroxylase & dopamine beta-hydroxylase mRNA levels in rat adrenals by a single & repeated immobilization stress. *J of Neurochemistry* 1992; 58(6):2124-30.
20 Salieva RM; et al. Delta sleep-inducing peptide as a factor increasing the content of substance P in the hypothalamus & the resistance of rats to emotional stress. *Neurosci & Beh Res* 1992 Jul-Aug; 22:275.
21 Kiseleva ZM. [Effect of emotional stress on catecholamine & dopa levels in some central nervous regions & in the heart of experimental animals]. *Kardiologiia* 1992 May; 32(5):81-4.
22 deCatanzaro D; Macniven E. Psychogenic pregnancy disruptions in mammals. *Neuroscience & Biobehavioral Revs* 1992 Spring; 16(1):43-53.

Chapter 14

1 Dalton, KD, *Once a Month* (Pomona, CA: Hunter House, 1979), p 178.
2 Wiklund I; et al. Long-term effect of transdermal hormonal therapy on aspects of quality of life in postmenopausal women. *Maturitas* 1992 Mar; 14(3):225-36.
3 Robert Atkins, M.D. Personal interview, January 29, 1993.
4 Lauersen NH. *Natural Progesterone* (New York).
5 Lee JR. Osteoporosis reversal with trnasdermal progesterone. *Lancet* 1990; 336:1327.
6 Lee JR. Is natural progesterone the missing link in osteoporosis prevention & treatment? *Med Hypothesis* 1991; 35:316-18.
7 Op cit, Dalton.
8 Colditz GA; et al. Type of postmenopausal hormone use & risk of breast cancer: 12-year follow-up from the Nurses' Health Study. *Cancer Causes & Control* 1992 Sep; 3(5):433-9.
9 Personal communication, Dr. Lee.
10 Letter from Esther M. Kirk, MD, Westwood Village, November 1984.
11 Letter from Louis J. Marx. MD, March 1984.
12 Richard Kunin, M.D. Personal communication, February 1, 1993.
13 Letter from John R. Lee, MD, April 1984.
14 Storch M; Carmichael C. *How to Relieve Cramps & other Menstrual Problems* (NY: Workman Publishing, 1982), p 49.
15 Dalton K. Prenatal Progesterone & Educational Attainments. *British J of Psychiatry* 1976; 129:438-42.
16 Reinisch JM; Ziemba-Davis M; Sanders SA. Hormonal contributions to sexually dimorphic behavioral development in humans. *PsychoneuroEnd* 1991; 16(1-3):213-78.
17 Foresta C; et al. Progesterone induces capacitation in human spermatozoa. *Andrologia* 1992; 24:33-5.
18 Ben-Nun I; et al. Therapeutic maturation of endometrium in in vitro fertilization & embryo transfer. *Fertility & Sterility* 1992 May; 57(5):953-62.
19 National Geographic, October 1992. Lee, John, MD. Personal interview, February 11, 1993.
20 Giamarchi D; et al. [Bronchial hyperreactivity in non-asthmatic patients harboring a uterine fibroma]. *Allergie et Immunologie* 1989 Feb; 21(2):72-5.
21 Dalton, KD, *Once a Month* (Pomona, CA, Hunter House, 1979), p 53.
22 Herzog AG. Reproductive endocrine considerations & hormonal therapy for women with epilepsy. *Epilepsia* 1991; 32 Suppl 6:S27-323 Tauboll E; Lindstrom S. The effect of progesterone & its metabolite

23 Tauboll E. Lindstrom S. The effect of progesterone & its metabolite 5 alpha-pregnan-3 alpha-ol-20-one on focal epileptic seizures in the cat's visual cortex in vivo. *Epilepsy Res* 1993 Jan; 14(1):17-30.

24 Lee, John, MD. Personal communication. Letter, December 11, 1992.

25 Hargrove JT; et al. Menopausal hormone replacement therapy with continuous daily oral micronized estradiol & progesterone. *Obstetrics & Gynecology* 1989; 73:606-12.

26 Wu ZY; Wu XK; Zhang YW. Relationship of menopausal status & sex hormones to serum lipids & blood pressure. *International J of Epidemiology* 1990 Jun; 19(2):297-302.

27 Crane Mg; Harris JJ; Winsor W II. Hypertension, oral contraceptive agents, & conjugated estrogen. *Annals of Int Med* 1971; 74:13-21.

28 Robert Atkins, MD. Personal interview, January 29, 1993.

29 Riis BJ; et al. The effect of percutaneous estradiol & natural progesterone on postmenopausal bone loss. *Amer J of Obstetrics & Gynecology* 1987; 156:61-5.

30 Steingold KA; et al. Comparison of transdermal to oral estradiol administration on hormonal & hepatic parameters in women with premature ovarian failure. *J of Clin End & Met* 1991 Aug; 73(2):275-80.

31 *Drugs* 1990.

32 *NEJM* 1989.

33 Ibid.

34 Segal S; Casper RF. Progesterone supplementation increases luteal phase endometrial thickness and estradiol levels in in-vitro fertilization. *Human Reproduction* 1992 Oct; 7(9):1210-13.

35 *Medical Hypothesis,* 1990.

36 Shaaban MM. Contraception with progestogens & progesterone during lactation. *J of Steroid Biochemistry & Molecular Biology* 1991; 40(4-6):705-10.

37 Norman RJ et al. Inhibin & relaxin concentrations in early singleton, multiple, & failing pregnancy: relationship to gonadotropin & steroid profiles. *Fertility & Sterility* Jan; 59(1):130-7.

38 Segal S; Casper RF. Progesterone supplementation increases luteal phase endometrial thickness & oestradiol levels in in-vitro fertilization. *Human Reproduction* 1992 Oct; 7(9):1210-3.

39 Laurikka-Routti M; Haukkamaa M; Lahteenmaki P. Suppression of ovarian function with the transder mally given synthetic progestin ST 1435. *Fertility & Sterility* 1992 Oct; 58(4):680-4.

40 Baird DT. Clin use of mifepristone (RU 486). *Annals of Med* 1993 Feb; 25(1):65-9.

41 Elks ML. Peripheral effects of sex steroids: implications for patient management. *J of the Amer Med Womens Assoc,* 1993 Mar-Apr, 48(2):41-6, 50.

42 Sitruk-Ware R. Percutaneous & transdermal ERT. *Annals of Med* 1993 Feb; 25(1):77-82.

43 Ibid.

44 Ibid.

45 Sitruk-Ware R. Estrogen therapy during menopause. Practical treatment recommendations. *Drugs,* 1990 Feb, 39(2):203-17.

46 Jordan VC; et al. The estrogenic activity of synthetic progestins used in oral contraceptives. *Cancer* 1993 Feb 15; 71(4 Suppl):1501-5.

Chapter 15

1 Baker DP. Estrogen-replacement therapy in patients with previous endometrial carcinoma. *Comprehen sive Therapy* 1990 Jan; 16(1):28-35.

2 Willett WC et al. Intake of *trans* fatty acids & risk of coronary heart disease. *Lancet* 1993; 341:581-5.

3 Froom J. Selections from current literature: hormone therapy in postmenopausal women. *Family Practice* 1991 Sep; 8(3):288-92.

4 Schlemmer A; et al. Urinary magnesium in early postmenopausal women. Influence of hormone therapy on calcium. *Magnesium & Trace Elements* 1991-92; 10(1):34-9.

5 Henderson BE; Bernstein L. The international variation in breast cancer rates: an epidemiological assessment. *Breast Cancer Res & Treatment* 1991 May; 18 Suppl 1:S11-7.

6 Cummings SR. Evaluating the benefits & risks of postmenopausal hormone therapy. *Amer J of Med* 1991 Nov 25; 91(5B):14S-18S.

7 Steingold KA; et al. Comparison of transdermal to oral estradiol administration on hormonal & hepatic parameters in women with premature ovarian failure. *J of Clin End & Met* 1991 Aug; 73(2):275-80.

8 Balfour JA; Heel RC. Transdermal estradiol. A Rev of its pharmacodynamic & pharmacokinetic properties, & therapeutic efficacy in the treatment of menopausal complaints. *Drugs* 1990 Oct; 40:561.

9 Wiklund I; et al. Long-term effect of transdermal hormonal therapy on aspects of quality of life in postmenopausal women. *Maturitas* 1992 Mar; 14(3):225-36.

10 Kirkham C; et al. A randomized, double-blind, placebo-controlled, cross-over trial to assess the side effects of medroxyprogesterone acetate in hormone replacement therapy. *O & Gyn* 1991 Jul; 78(1):93-7.

11 Testimony presented to FDAs Fertility & Maternal Health Drugs Advisory Committee, June, 1992.

12 Ibid.

13 Cundy T. *British Med J* 1991 July 6.

14 Stehlin D. Depo-provera: the quarterly contraceptive. *FDA Consumer* 1993; 27:11-13.

15 Metzger DA; et al. Are estrogens indicated for the treatment of postmenopausal women? *Drugs.*

16 Backstrom T; et al. PMS—psychiatric or gynaecological disorder? *Ann of Med* 1991 Dec; 23(6):625-33.

17 Ibid.

18 Leather AT; et al. Endometrial histology & bleeding patterns after 8 years of continuous combined estrogen & progestogen therapy in postmenopausal women.*Obstetrics & Gynecology* 1991Dec; 78(6):1008.

19 Op cit, Wikland.

20 Amano K; et al. [Effect of suppletory estrogen or 1,25(OH)D3 on bone mineral content.] *Acta Obstetrica et Gynaecologica Japonica* 1992 Jul; 44(7):83.

21 Wolf PH; et al. Reduction of cardiovascular disease-related mortality among postmenopausal women who use hormones. *Amer J of Obstetrics & Gynecology* 1991 Feb; 164(2):489-94.

22 Konner M. *Med at the Crossroads* (New York: Pantheon Books, 1993), p 75.

23 Schneider HP; Doren M. [Osteoporosis from the gynecologic viewpoint]. *Zentralblatt fur Gynakologie* 1992; 114(7):333-50.

24 Baum E. [Psychosocial effects of the onset of menopause & physical symptoms in early postmenopause]. *Psychotherapie, Psychosomatik, Medizinische Psychologie,* 1990 Jun; 40(6):200-6.

25 Ferguson KJ; et al. Estrogen replacement therapy. A survey. *Archives of Int Med*, 1989 Jan; 149(1):133.

26 Spicer DV; et al. Sex steroids and breast cancer prevention. *Monographs*/National Cancer Institute 1994; (16):139-47.

27 Schlemmer A; et al. Urinary magnesium in early postmenopausal women. Influence of hormone therapy on calcium. *Magnesium & Trace Elements*, 1991-92; 10(1):34-9.

28 Reinisch JM; Ziemba-Davis M; Sanders SA. Hormonal contributions to sexually dimorphic behavioral development in humans. *Psychoneuroendocrinology*, 1991; 16(1-3):213-78.

29 Doren M; Schneider HP. Identification & treatment of postmenopausal women at risk for the development of osteoporosis. *Int J of Clin Pharmacology, Therapy, & Toxicology*, 1992 Nov; 30; (11):431-3.

30 Lindsay R. The effect of sex steroids on the skeleton in premenopausal women. *Amer J of Obs & Gyn*, 1992 Jun; 166(6 Pt 2):1993-6.

30 Lindsay R. Effect of sex steroids on skeleton. *Amer J of Ob & Gyn*, Jun 1992; 166(6 Pt 2):1993-6.

31 Sitruk-Ware R. Percutaneous & transdermal ert. *Annals of Med*, Feb 1993; 25(1):77-82.

32 VanVollenhoven RF; et al. Estrogten, progesterone, and testosterone; can they be used to t6reat autoimmune diseases? *Clev Clin J Med* 1994; 61(4):276-84.

33 Rozenberg S; et al. Decrease of bone mineral density during estrogen substitution therapy.*Maturitas* 1993; 17(3):205-10.

34 Op cit, Lindsey.

35 Jordan VC; et al. The estrogenic activity of synthetic progestins used in oral contraceptives. *Cancer*, 1993 Feb15; 71(4 Suppl):1501-5.

36 Felson DT; et al. Effect of postmenopausal ERT on bone density in elderly women.*NEJM* 1993; 329:1141.

37 Ibid.

38 Nordon BE; et al. The relative contribution of age & years since menopause to postmenopausal bone loss. *J of Clin End Met* 1990; 70:83-88.

39 Heany RP. Estrogen-calcium interactions in the postmenopause: a quantitative description.*Bone Mineral* 1990; 11:67-84.

40 Eisenberg DM; et al. Unconventional Med in the United States: prevavlennce, costs, & patterns of use. *NEJM* 1993; 328:246-52.

AFTERWORD

1 *British Medical Journal* 1994 May 14; 1268-69.

2 Editorial. *Lancet* 1995; 345:933-935.

3 Commentary. *Lancet* 1995; 345:876.

4 Ibid.

5 Cummings SR. Risk factors for hip fracture in white women. *NEJM* 1995; 332:767-773.

6 Federman DD. Life without estrogen. *NEJM* 1994; 331:1088-89.

7 Dwyer Jt; et al. Tofu and soy drinks contain phytoestrogens. *J Am Diet Assoc* 1994; 94:739-43.

8 Rhoades R; Pflanzer R. *Human Physiology*. (NY: Harcourt Brace, Saunders College Publishing, 1992).

INDEX